Low Risk Neonatal Nurse Exam Part 2 of 2

SECRETS

Study Guide
Your Key to Exam Success

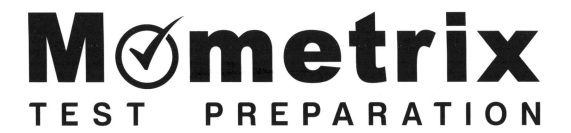

DEAR FUTURE EXAM SUCCESS STORY

First of all, **THANK YOU** for purchasing Mometrix study materials!

Second, congratulations! You are one of the few determined test-takers who are committed to doing whatever it takes to excel on your exam. **You have come to the right place.** We developed these study materials with one goal in mind: to deliver you the information you need in a format that's concise and easy to use.

In addition to optimizing your guide for the content of the test, we've outlined our recommended steps for breaking down the preparation process into small, attainable goals so you can make sure you stay on track.

We've also analyzed the entire test-taking process, identifying the most common pitfalls and showing how you can overcome them and be ready for any curveball the test throws you.

Standardized testing is one of the biggest obstacles on your road to success, which only increases the importance of doing well in the high-pressure, high-stakes environment of test day. Your results on this test could have a significant impact on your future, and this guide provides the information and practical advice to help you achieve your full potential on test day.

Your success is our success

We would love to hear from you! If you would like to share the story of your exam success or if you have any questions or comments in regard to our products, please contact us at **800-673-8175** or **support@mometrix.com**.

Thanks again for your business and we wish you continued success!

Sincerely,
The Mometrix Test Preparation Team

> **Need more help? Check out our flashcards at:**
> **http://mometrixflashcards.com/Neonatal**

TABLE OF CONTENTS

General Management (Continued)

Pharmacology, Pharmacokinetics, and Pharmacodynamics

PRINCIPLES OF PHARMACOKINETICS

Pharmacokinetics relates to the route of administration, the absorption, the dosage, the frequency of administration, the distribution, and the serum levels achieved over time. The drug's *rate of clearance* (elimination) and doses needed to ensure therapeutic benefit must be considered. Most drugs are cleared through the kidneys, with water-soluble compounds excreted more readily than protein-soluble compounds. *Volume of distribution* (IV drug dose divided by plasma concentration) determines the rate at which the drug passes into tissue. Drug distribution depends on the degree of protein binding and ion trapping that takes place.

Elimination half-life is the time needed to reduce plasma concentrations to 50% during elimination. Approximately five half-lives are needed to achieve steady-state plasma concentrations if giving doses intermittently. *Context-sensitive half-life* is the time needed to reach 50% concentration after withdrawal of a continuously-administered drug. *Recovery time* is the length of time it takes for plasma levels to decrease to the point that the effect is eliminated. This is affected by plasma concentration. *Effect-site equilibrium* is the time between administration of a drug and clinical effect (the point at which the drug reaches the appropriate receptors) and must be considered when determining dose, time, and frequency of medications. The *bioavailability* of drugs may vary, depending upon the degree of metabolism that takes place before the drug reaches its site of action.

PRINCIPLES OF PHARMACODYNAMICS

Pharmacodynamics relates to biological effects (therapeutic or adverse) of drug administration over time. Drug transport, absorption, means of elimination, and half-life must all be considered when determining effects. Responses may include continuous responses, such as blood pressure variations, or dichotomous response in which an event either occurs or does not (such as death). Information from pharmacodynamics provides feedback to modify medication dosage (pharmacokinetics). Drugs provide biological effects primarily by interacting with receptor sites (specific protein molecules) in the cell membrane. Receptors include voltage-sensitive ion channels (sodium, chloride, potassium, and calcium channels), ligand-gated ion channels, and transmembrane receptors. Agonist drugs exert effects after binding with a receptor while antagonist drugs bind with a receptor but have no effects, so they can block agonists from binding. The total number of receptors may vary, upregulating or downregulating in response to stimuli (such as drug administration). Dose-response curves show the relationship between the amount of drug given and the resultant plasma concentration and biological effects.

PRINCIPLES OF ADMINISTRATION

DOSAGE AND INTERVAL

The half-life of a drug ($t_{1/2}$) is the time required to reduce serum concentrations by half, and half-life must be considered when determining **dosage and interval** of drugs for neonates. Steady state is usually achieved within 4 to 5 half-lives. Half-life is a factor of clearance, and small or preterm infants often have reduced clearance because of slow metabolism, resulting in longer half-life. In

1

determining dosage, the infant's weight, gestational age, as well as post-natal age must be considered. Relevant formulas include:

- T ½ = 0.7 x Volume of distribution/Clearance.
- Loading dose = (Volume of distribution x concentration)/ F.

One major problem with dosing and interval for neonates is that most drugs are not tested on infants, so about 98% are prescribed off-label. There are a number of reference tools available, including software programs, to assist with determining proper dosage and interval for neonatal medications.

TOLERANCE AND WEANING

Tolerance and weaning from drugs are most often concerns with administration of opiates. Tolerance occurs after repeated administration results in a lessoning of effects, requiring an increase in dosage to achieve the same results. When a neonate is weaned from a medication or a dosage is decreased, only one class of medications should be involved. Thus, if the infant is receiving both an opiate and a benzodiazepine, they should not be weaned at the same time. The infant should be evaluated for level of pain prior to weaning and the reassessed at least every 4 hours during the weaning process. Usually medications are reduced at a rate of 10% per day or 20% every other day. Infants often tolerate an initial reduction in dose better than subsequent reductions, so careful observation for signs of increased pain or withdrawal must be made. Careful control of the environment—temperature, light, and noise—should be done to reduce infant stress during the weaning process.

DRUG INTERACTIONS

Drug interactions occur when one drug interferes with the activity of another in either the pharmacodynamics or pharmacokinetics:

- With **pharmacodynamic interaction,** both drugs may interact at receptor sites causing a change that results in an adverse effect or that interferes with a positive effect.
- With **pharmacokinetic interaction**, the ability of the drug to be absorbed and cleared is altered, so there may be delayed effects, changes in effects, or toxicity. Interactions may include problems in a number of areas:
  - **Absorption** may be increased or (more commonly) decreased, usually related to the effects within the gastrointestinal system.
  - **Distribution** of drugs may be affected, often because of changes in protein binding.
  - **Metabolism** may be altered, often causing changes in drug concentration.
  - **Biotransformation** of the drug must take place, usually in the liver and gastrointestinal system, but drug interactions can impair this process.
  - **Clearance interactions** may interfere with the body's ability to eliminate a drug, usually resulting in increased concentration of the drug.

PROTEIN BINDING

Protein binding is an important consideration for neonatal drug therapy because when drugs are bound by proteins in the blood, they are not available to be biologically active. The portion of the

2

drug that is **not** bound to a plasma protein is the active portion. Protein binding is significant in premature neonates because they typically have:

- Lower levels of plasma proteins, such as albumin.
- Lower binding capacity.
- Susceptibility to competition from endogenous substances like bilirubin, which also attaches to plasma proteins.

Drugs that are normally highly protein bound in the adult have a higher free percentage (activity) in the neonate. Lower than expected dosages may give clinical results. Examples of drugs that are highly protein bound include Phenobarbital and Indomethacin. Is a drug with a high affinity for plasma proteins is administered, it may displace bilirubin from binding sites, increasing the neonate's risk for kernicterus.

FIRST PASS METABOLISM AND DRUG CLEARANCE

First pass metabolism: This is the phenomenon that occurs to ingested drugs that are absorbed through the gastrointestinal tract and enter the hepatic portal system. Drugs metabolized on the first pass travel to the liver, where they are broken down, some to the extent that only a small fraction of the active drug circulates to the rest of the body. This first pass through the liver greatly reduces the bioavailability of some drugs. Routes of administration that avoid first pass metabolism include intravenous, intramuscular, and sublingual.

Drug Clearance: This is the ability to remove a drug from the body. The two main organs responsible for clearance are the liver and the kidneys. The liver eliminates drugs by metabolizing, or biotransforming the substance, or excreting the drug in the bile. The kidneys eliminate drugs by filtration or active excretion in the urine. Drugs use either renal or hepatic methods of clearance. Kidney and liver dysfunction inhibit the clearance of drugs that rely on that organ for removal. Toxicity results from poor clearance.

ENTEROHEPATICALLY RECIRCULATED DRUGS AND RENALLY-EXCRETED DRUGS

Enterohepatically recirculated drugs are effectively removed from circulation and then reabsorbed. These drugs are secreted in bile, which is collected in the gall bladder and emptied into the small intestine, from which part of it is reabsorbed and part excreted in the feces. This reabsorption reduces the clearance of these drugs and increases their duration of action. Generally, drugs susceptible to enterohepatic recirculation are those with a molecular weight greater than 300 g/mole and those that are amphipathic (have both a lipophilic portion and a polar portion).

Renally-excreted drugs are metabolized (biotransformed) by the liver to a form that can be excreted by the kidneys. Others are excreted by the kidneys unchanged. Infants with decreased renal function demonstrate decreased urine output or elevated levels of BUN and creatinine. The nurse should avoid using drugs that depend on the kidneys for clearance if the infant has renal impairment as overdose may result.

FORMULAS FOR ABSORPTION, DISTRIBUTION, AND CLEARANCE

Absorption: This relates to the rate at which a drug enters the blood stream and the amount of drug.

F = the percentage of a drug's availability for absorption (with 1 equal to 100%).

Distribution: The volume of distribution is the relationship between the total loading dose of drug administered and the serum concentration. (Volume of body fluid required to dissolve the amount of drug found in the serum). This is usually expressed as units of volume per kg of weight:

Loading dose x F = Change in concentration x volume of distribution.

Clearance: Elimination pathways (liver, kidney) can become saturated if dose of medications is too high or administration is too frequent. Ideally, a drug concentration should be maintained at a steady state (average):

Clearance = F x Dose/dose interval x steady stage concentration.

Dose rate = (Clearance x steady state concentration)/ F.

PLACENTAL TRANSFER OF DRUGS

The **placenta** acts as a barrier to protect the fetus, but its main function is to provide oxygen and nutrients for the fetus by linking the maternal and fetal circulation. Virtually all **drugs** cross the barrier to some degree, some by active transport. Some drugs are readily diffused across the placental barrier and can affect the fetus. Drugs that are non-ionized, fat-soluble and have low molecular weight diffuse easily as glucose does. Once a substance crosses the barrier, the lower pH of the fetal blood allows weakly basic drugs, such as local anesthetics and opioids, to cross into fetal circulation where they become ionized and accumulate because they can't pass back into maternal circulation (ion trapping). Giving an intravenous injection during a contraction, when uterine blood flow decreases, reduces the amount of the drug that crosses the placental barrier. A few drugs with large molecules (heparin, insulin) have minimal transfer, and lipid soluble drugs transfer more readily than water-soluble.

ROUTES OF MEDICATION ADMINISTRATION

The absorption rate of a drug depends on its transfer from its site of administration to the circulatory system. Different **routes of administration** have different absorption characteristics:

- **Oral**: Ingested medications pass from the gastrointestinal tract into the blood stream. Most absorption occurs in the small intestine and is affected by gastric motility and emptying rate, drug solubility in gastrointestinal fluids, and food presence. Orally administered drugs are susceptible to first pass metabolism by the liver.
- **Intravenous**: Medications directly administered to the blood stream have 100% absorption. Peak serum levels are rapidly achieved. Some drugs are not tolerated intravenously, due to vein irritation or toxicity, and others must be given as an infusion.
- **Intramuscular**: Medications injected into a muscle are fairly rapidly absorbed because muscle tissue is highly vascularized. Drugs in lipid vehicles absorb more slowly than those in aqueous vehicles.
- **Subcutaneous**: Medications injected beneath the skin absorb more slowly because the dermis is less vascularized than muscle. Hypoperfusion and edema decrease absorption further.

5 RIGHTS OF MEDICATION ADMINISTRATION

The **5 rights of medication administration** are used to prevent/reduce medication errors in the hospital setting. Often these 5 rights are integrated into the scanning requirements of electronic documentation. The 5 rights of medication administration must also be incorporated into the prescriber's order:

- **Right Patient**: Confirm the patient's identity using two identifiers, often being their full name and date of birth. Scanning will also confirm the patient's identity with their bar code and electronic health record.
- **Right Drug**: Check the name of the drug with the prescriber's order. By scanning the medication, the drug name will also be checked against the order.
- **Right Dose**: Check the dose of the drug with the prescriber's order. Some medications require a second nurse confirm any dosage calculations utilized before administration. Ensure the dosage is appropriate and contact the prescriber if there are any concerns.
- **Right route**: Routes include oral (PO), subcutaneous, intradermal, IV, or IM, amongst others. The route must also be confirmed with the prescriber's order.
- **Right time/frequency**: The drug may be administered as a one-time dose, PRN (as needed), or recurring administration (twice daily, every 8 hours, etc.).

BLOOD DRUG LEVELS

Plasma drug levels are used for **therapeutic drug monitoring** because, although plasma is often not the site of action, plasma levels correlate well with therapeutic (effective) and toxic (dose-related adverse effects) responses to most drugs. The therapeutic range of a drug is that between the minimum effective concentration (level at which there is no therapeutic benefit) and the toxic concentration (level at which toxic effects occur). To achieve drug plateau (steady state), the drug half-life (time needed to decrease drug concentration by 50%) must be considered. Most drugs reach plateau with administration equal to four half-lives and completely eliminate a drug in 5 half-lives. Because drug levels fluctuate, peak (highest drug concentration) and trough (lowest drug concentration) levels may be monitored. Samples for trough levels are taken immediately prior to administration of another dose while peak samples are taken at various times, depending on the average peak time of the specific drug, which may vary from 30 minutes to 2 hours or so after administration.

ANTICOAGULANTS

Neonates may require **anticoagulant therapy** for thrombosis, sometimes associated with catheters used for critical care or thrombocytosis associated with iron-deficiency anemia. Anticoagulant therapy poses fewer risks than fibrinolytic therapy although excessive bleeding may occur. Anticoagulants include:

- **Unfractionated heparin:**
  - Preterm infants: Initial bolus of 50 units/kg and maintenance of 15 units to 35 units/kg/hr to maintain level of 0.3 to 0.7 units/mL.
  - Full-term infants: Initial bolus of 100 units/kg and maintenance of 25 units to 50 units/kg/hr to maintain level of 0.3 to 0.7 unit/mL.
- **Low-molecular-weight heparin:** 1.7 mg/kg sq every 12 hours or as needed to maintain level of 0.5 to 1 units/ml 4 hours after administration.
- **Warfarin:** May be used in rare cases, such as genetic deficiencies of protein C or S (purpura fulminans), for long-term therapy.

Infants that are heparin resistant may be administered fresh frozen plasma (1 mL/kg every 24-48 hours) or AT concentrate (50-150 units/kg every 24-48 hours) to enhance effect of heparin.

ANTICONVULSANTS

Anticonvulsants are used to treat seizures, which often indicate central nervous system dysfunction. Seizures are more common during the neonatal period than later in infancy/childhood and are associated with low birth weight. Treatment is critical to prevent brain damage, but drugs may cause sedation, rash, and blood dyscrasias:

- **Phenobarbital** (Luminal®) is the neonatal drug of choice. Loading dose is 20 mg/kg IV in 10-15 minutes and then 5 mg/kg to maximum 40 mg/kg to control seizures. Maintenance dose is 3 to 4 mg /kg/24 hours in 2 doses beginning ≥12 hours after loading dose. Infant should be provided oxygen and ventilation as needed.
- **Fosphenytoin** (Cerbxy®) is used if phenobarbital is ineffective. It has high water solubility and neutral pH and does not cause tissue injury. It can be administered IV or IM. Loading dose is 15 to 20mgPE/kg and maintenance id 4 to 8mg PE/kg/24 hrs. Blood pressure should be monitored and caution exercised with hyperbilirubinemia. (Continued)
- **Phenytoin** (Dilantin®) is sometimes used instead of fosphenytoin if phenobarbital is ineffective. It is incompatible with other drugs and glucose and can cause hypotension, bradycardia, and dysrhythmias if administered too quickly and cannot be given IM or in central lines. Loading dose is 15-20 mg/kg IV over 30 minutes, and maintenance is 4-8 mg/kg/24 hours. Line must be flushed with NS.
- **Lorazepam** (Ativan®) is used if other drugs are ineffective in controlling seizures. Onset is action is very rapid (<5 minutes), so the infant must be monitored carefully for respiratory depression. Medication is administered by slow IV push over a number of minutes at 0.05 to 0.1 mg/kg.

In some cases, seizures are triggered by hypoglycemia, and treatment includes glucose 10% solution. Pyridoxine (B_6) deficiency may also cause seizures and is treated with IV or IM Vitamin B_6.

GENTAMICIN

Gentamicin is an inexpensive aminoglycoside antibiotic commonly used to treat neonates with gram-negative bacterial infections, like *Staphylococci*. It works by interfering with bacterial protein synthesis, resulting in a defective bacterial cell membrane. Gentamicin is excreted unmetabolized by the kidneys and renal function is directly related to clearance. Clearance is slower in premature neonates secondary to immature kidneys. The peak level (highest concentration in the blood) of gentamicin is measured 30 minutes after infusion is completed, and trough level (lowest concentration of the drug in the blood) is measured 30 minutes prior to the next dose. Potential toxicities from elevated gentamicin levels are ototoxicity (ear damage potentiated by concurrent use of furosemide) and nephrotoxicity (kidney damage), so patients with renal failure may only require dosing once every several days. If the pre-dose level falls below 0.5 mg/L and the post-dose level falls below 4 mg/L, the gentamicin is sub-therapeutic and will not kill the bacterial infection.

ANTIBIOTICS

Antimicrobials include antibiotics, antifungals, and antivirals. **Antibiotics** may be classified according to their chemical nature, origin, action, or range of effectiveness. **Broad-spectrum antibiotics** are useful against both gram-positive and gram-negative bacteria. **Medium-spectrum antibiotics** are usually effective against gram-positive bacteria, although some may also be effective against gram-negative bacteria. **Narrow-spectrum antibiotics** are effective against a small range of bacteria. Antibiotics kill the bacteria by interfering with their biological functions

6

(bacteriocidal) or by preventing reproduction (bacteriostatic). The main classes of antibiotics include the following:

- **Macrolides:** Medium-spectrum antibiotics
- **Penicillins:** Medium-spectrum antibiotics, may be combined with beta-lactamase inhibitors; may cause severe allergic reactions
- **Cephalosporins:** Medium-spectrum antibiotics effective against gram-negative organisms
- **Polymyxins:** Narrow-spectrum antibiotics effective against gram-negative organisms
- **Fluoroquinolones:** Broad-spectrum antibiotics
- **Sulfonamides:** Medium-spectrum antibiotics with action against gram-positive and many gram-negative organisms, as well as Plasmodium and Toxoplasma
- **Tetracyclines:** Broad-spectrum antibiotics (can cause mottling/discoloration of later teeth)
- **Aminoglycosides:** Effective against gram-negative bacteria

NEONATAL ANTI-VIRAL DRUGS

Acyclovir	IV: 60 mg/kg/d x 14-21 days	Indicated for herpes simples and varicella zoster infections. Complications include rash, TTP, hemolytic uremic syndrome, increased liver enzymes, urea, and creatinine.
Ganciclovir	IV: 6 mg/kg q 12 hr X 6 weeks	Indicated for cytomegalovirus (disseminated, pneumonia). Complications include neutropenia, thrombocytopenia, phlebitis, rash, increased liver function tests, seizures.
Palivizumab (Synagis®)	IV or IM: 15 mg/kg monthly during season or while at risk.	Humanized monoclonal antibody indicated to treat or protect against respiratory syncytial virus for neonates with severe respiratory disease, such as bronchopulmonary dysplasia. Complications include fever, poor feeding, bleeding, irritability, wheezing, allergic reaction.
Respiratory Syncytial Virus Immune Globulin (RSVIG/RespiGam®)	IV: 750 mg/kg (15 mL/kg) with slow infusion.	Indicated for prophylaxis against respiratory syncytial virus but less potent than palivizumab and requires IV administration and larger volume. Complications include fever, wheezing, GI upset, allergic reaction, muscle rigidity.

ANTI-HYPERTENSIVES AND OTHER CARDIAC DRUGS

Antihypertensives are used to control congestive heart failure and reduce the cardiac workload:

- **Captopril** is an ace inhibitor is used to control hypertension.
- **Propranolol** is a beta-blocker used to control hypertension.
- **Labetalol** (Normodyne®, Trandate®) is an alpha-1 and beta-adrenergic blocker that slows the heart rate and decreases peripheral vascular resistance and cardiac output.

Miscellaneous cardiac drugs are used for specific purposes:

- **Calcium chloride/Calcium gluconate** is given intravenously after surgery to increase myocardial contractibility.
- **Brevibloc** (Esmolol®) is a beta-blocker given intravenously after surgery to control systemic hypertension, arrhythmias, and outflow obstruction.

7

- **Indomethacin** (Indocin®) is a NSAID that is given intravenously to inhibit the production of prostaglandin, thereby speeding the closure of the ductus arteriosus.
- **Prostaglandin** is given intravenously before surgery to maintain the patency of the ductus arteriosus for structural cardiac abnormalities in conditions such as coarctation of the aorta or transposition of the great arteries.

DIURETICS

Diuretics are used in the cardiac patient to increase renal perfusion and filtration, thereby reducing preload. Dosages are weight and age related. Diuretics commonly used include:

- **Bumetanide** (Bumex®) is a loop diuretic (acting on the renal ascending loop of Henle) given intravenously after surgery to reduce preload.
- **Ethacrynic acid** (Edecrin®) is a loop diuretic given intravenously after surgery to reduce preload.
- **Furosemide** (Lasix®) is a loop diuretic and is used for the control of congestive heart failure as well as renal insufficiency. It is used after surgery to decrease preload and to reduce the inflammatory response caused by cardiopulmonary bypass (post-perfusion syndrome).
- **Spironolactone** (Aldactone®) is a potassium-sparing synthetic steroid diuretic that increases the secretion of both water and sodium and is used to treat congestive heart failure. It may be given orally or intravenously.

LOOP, THIAZIDE, AND POTASSIUM-SPARING DIURETICS

Diuretics decrease the fluid load in infants with heart failure or lung disorders, such as bronchopulmonary dysplasia. Different **classes of diuretics** have different mechanisms of action and different side effect profiles:

- **Loop diuretics** (e.g., furosemide) are the most potent of the diuretics and work on the ascending limb of the loop of Henle. They disrupt the Na+/K+/2Cl- transporter and also limit K+ reabsorption. Hypokalemia, hyponatremia, and increased calcium excretion are the adverse reactions seen with chronic use.
- **Thiazide diuretics** (e.g., chlorothiazide) work by inhibiting Na+/Cl- transport in the distal convoluted tubule. They are less potent than loop diuretics. Hyponatremia, hypokalemia, and hypomagnesemia are the adverse reactions from chronic use.
- **Potassium-sparing diuretics** (e.g., spironolactone) work by inhibiting the action of aldosterone. Aldosterone promotes K+ secretion and Na+ reabsorption at the distal nephron. These diuretics are the least potent, but do not cause hypokalemia.

VASODILATORS AND ANTI-ARRHYTHMICS

Vasodilators may be used for arterial dilation or venous dilation. These drugs are used to treat pulmonary hypertension or generalized systemic hypertension. Dosages are weight and age related. Vasodilators include:

- **Nitroglycerine** is used intravenously after surgery to improve myocardial perfusion by dilating the coronary arteries. It can be used as a venous dilator and decreases the diastolic pressure of the left ventricle and reduces systemic vascular resistance (SVR).
- **Nitroprusside** is given intravenously before and after surgery for peripheral vascular dilation to decrease afterload and SVR in order to increase cardiac output.

8

Anti-arrhythmics are used to control arrhythmias and slow the heart rate:

- **Amiodarone** is given intravenously after surgery to reduce AV and SA conduction, slowing the heartbeat. It is used to control both ventricular dysrhythmias and junctional ectopic tachycardia.
- **Lidocaine** is given intravenously before and after surgery to control ventricular dysrhythmias.
- **Procainamide** is given intravenously after surgery to control supraventricular tachycardia and is effective for both atrial and ventricular tachycardia.

VASOPRESSORS/INOTROPES

Drugs used to increase cardiac output and improve contractibility of the myocardium are the **vasopressors/inotropes**. Dosage and administration of pediatric medications is weight and age related. Inotropes include:

- **Dobutamine** is given intravenously before and after surgery to improve cardiac output and treat cardiac decompensation.
- **Dopamine** is given intravenously before and after surgery to increase cardiac output, blood pressure, and the excretion of urine.
- **Digoxin** is given intravenously or by mouth and is used to increase the strength of myocardial contractions, resulting in better cardiac output.
- **Epinephrine** is given intravenously before and after surgery to increase blood pressure and cardiac output, but it must be used judiciously because it also increases consumption of oxygen.
- **Milrinone/Amrinone** is given after surgery to increase cardiac output and stroke volume, decrease systemic vascular resistance (SVR) as well as control congestive heart failure.

DIGITALIS

Digitalis is a cardiac glycoside that is used to treat congestive heart failure (CHF) and several different cardiac arrhythmias. Digitalis slows and strengthens the heartbeat. It has both a direct action on the myocardium and an indirect action mediated through the autonomic nervous system. The direct effect on the myocardium works by inhibiting the action of the sodium/potassium pump across cardiac cell membranes. The net result is an increase in intracellular sodium and calcium and an increase in extracellular potassium. The intracellular calcium is responsible for the increased strength of contractions of the heart (positive ionotrope). The indirect action of digitalis causes the heart rate to slow (negative chronotrope) by decreasing electrical conduction through the AV node. Digoxin has a narrow therapeutic index, meaning the lethal dose is close to the therapeutic dose. Signs of **digitalis toxicity** in infants include:

- GI signs: Anorexia, nausea, vomiting, and diarrhea.
- Cardiac arrhythmias: Most commonly conduction disturbances, such as first-degree heart block, a supraventricular tachyarrhythmia such as atrial tachycardia, or bradycardia.

Assume any alteration in cardiac conduction in an infant taking digoxin is a consequence of digitalis toxicity.

VOLATILE ANESTHETICS

Small infants have a high water content (70-75%) compared to adults (50-60%), and a lower muscle mass. These factors, coupled with slow renal and hepatic clearance, increased rate of metabolism, decreased protein binding, and increased organ perfusion affect the pharmacological

9

action of drugs. Pediatric doses are calculated according to the child's weight in kilograms, but other factors may affect dosage. **Anesthetic agents** must be chosen with care because of the potential for adverse effects:

INHALATIONAL

Infants are more likely to develop hypotension and bradycardia with inhalational anesthetic agents. Inhalation induction is rapid because infants and young children have high alveolar ventilation and decreased FRC compared to older patients with depression of ventilation more common in infants. There is increased risk of overdose. Sevoflurane is usually preferred for induction and isoflurane or halothane for maintenance as desflurane and sevoflurane are associated with delirium on emergence.

NONVOLATILE ANESTHETICS

Infants may need higher proportionate (based on weight) doses of *propofol* because it is eliminated more quickly than with adults. It should not be used for infants who are critically ill, as it has been correlated to increased mortality rate and severe adverse effects leading to multi-organ failure. *Thiopental* also is used in higher proportionate doses for infants and children although this is not true for neonates. Neonates are especially sensitive to opioids, and *morphine* should be avoided or used with caution. Clearance rates for some drugs (sufentanil, alfentanil) may be higher in infants. *Ketamine* combined with *fentanyl* may cause more hypotension in neonates and small infants than ketamine combined with midazolam. *Midazolam* combined with fentanyl can cause severe hypotension. *Etomidate* is not used for infants but is reserved for children >10.

MUSCLE RELAXANTS

Onset with muscle relaxants is about 50% shorter in infants than adults, and pediatric patients may have variable responses to muscle to non-depolarizing muscle relaxants. Drugs that are metabolized through the liver (pancuronium, vecuronium, and cisatracurium) have prolonged action, so atracurium and cisatracurium, which do not depend on the liver, are more reliable. Succinylcholine can cause severe adverse effects (rhabdomyolysis, malignant hyperthermia, hyperkalemia, arrhythmias), so its use requires premedication with atropine, but succinylcholine is usually avoided in pediatric patients except for rapid sequence induction for children with full stomach and laryngospasm. Rocuronium is frequently used for intubation because of fast onset, but it has up to 90 minutes duration, so mivacurium, atracurium, and cisatracurium may be preferred for shorter procedures. Nerve stimulators should be used to monitor incremental doses, which are usually 25-30% of the original bolus. Blockade by non-depolarizing muscle relaxants can be reversed with neostigmine or edrophonium and glycopyrrolate or atropine.

BRONCHODILATORS AND RESPIRATORY STIMULANTS

Bronchodilators and respiratory stimulants are used to treat respiratory distress in the neonate:

- **Aminophylline and theophylline** both stimulate the sympathetic nervous system and dilate the bronchi. These medications are used for apnea of prematurity in the neonate and bronchospasm in infants with respiratory distress. Apnea of prematurity is treated with loading dose of 6 mg/kg aminophylline with maintenance doses of 2.5-3.5 mg/kg intravenously every 12 hours. Further treatment may be done orally with theophylline. Side effects include tachycardia, seizures, and irritability.
- **Albuterol** is a selective β2-adrenergic agonist bronchodilator that can be administered orally (100-300 µg/kg 3-4 times daily) or inhaled (100-500 µg/kg 4-8 times daily).

- **Caffeine citrate,** a stimulant, is the first line treatment for apnea of prematurity as it is safer than theophylline and can be administered orally. Loading dose is usually 20 mg/mg with one-time daily maintenance dose of 5mg/kg.
- **Epinephrine** is used to treat stridor with effect on β-adrenoreceptors. It is delivered with nebulizer at 50-100 µg/kg as needed.

CAFFEINE FOR NEONATAL APNEA

Apnea of prematurity occurs when the neonate stops breathing for 20 seconds or longer because the respiratory centers are immature. Apnea of prematurity is an exclusionary diagnosis, arrived at only when all other causes have been ruled out. Treatment consists of respiratory support with supplemental oxygen, continuous positive airway pressure (CPAP), or a ventilator in severe cases. **Caffeine** has largely replaced theophylline as the pharmacological treatment of choice for apnea of prematurity. Both are methylxanthines, but caffeine has a wider therapeutic index and a slower excretion rate than theophylline. Caffeine is a **central nervous system stimulant** that naturally occurs in tea, coffee, and chocolate. Give 10 mg CAFCIT to the infant orally. Side effects include: Irritability; tremors; tachycardia; tachypnea; vomiting; fever; and hyperglycemia. Peak blood levels will be reached in 30 minutes-2 hours and should not exceed 6-10 mg/L. Toxicity is 50 mg/L. If seizures occur with caffeine overdose, give diazepam or pentobarbital sodium. Mean half-life is 3-4 days. Monitor trough levels periodically.

SURFACTANTS

Surfactants reduce surface tension to prevent collapse of alveoli. Beractant (Survanta®) is derived from bovine lung tissue and calfactant (Infasurf®) from calf lung tissue. Surfactant replacement therapy is used to prevent RDS for infants born at 27-30 weeks gestation. It is also used for infants showing signs of worsening lung disease. Surfactant is given via the endotracheal tube (ETT) as an inhalant. All four lung fields are coated with surfactant, so the dose is roughly divided into four equal parts. The head of the bed is declined to put the baby in a head down position. The head is turned to one direction, and the first dose is put down the ETT. To reach the other upper lung field, the head is turned the other direction, and the second dose given vial the ETT. Once the upper lung fields have received their doses, the head of the bed is inclined to reach the lower fields. The head turning procedure is repeated until all four doses have been given.

STEROIDS

Steroids are commonly administered to mothers to promote fetal lung development for preterm births. These drugs include betamethasone and dexamethasone. Steroids may also be administered to the neonate, but they are associated with significant side effects:

- **Betamethasone** may be used for chronic lung disease (CLD) in the neonate and post-intubation airway edema, but high dose treatment has been associated with cerebral palsy, growth depression, hypertension, hyperglycemia, hypokalemia, and increased risk of infection. Airway edema is treated with 200 µg/kg orally/IV every 8 hours beginning 4 hours before extubation. Dosages for other treatment vary widely with tapering of doses.
- **Hydrocortisone** may be used for physiologic replacement or acute hypotension. Replacement is begun with 1-2 mg orally every 8 hours and increased to 6-9 mg/m2/day. Hypotension is treated with 2 mg/kg IV loading dose and maintenance of 1 mg/kg IV every 8-12 hours.

VITAMIN K DEFICIENCY

Vitamin K deficiency in newborns may cause vitamin K deficiency bleeding (VKDB), also called **hemorrhagic disease of the newborn**. Vitamin K is a fat-soluble vitamin produced in the gut.

Vitamin K is required by the liver to produce four of the clotting factors—II, VII, IX, and X. At birth, all infants are Vitamin K deficient because of limited transfer of vitamin K across the placenta. Newborns are injected with intramuscular vitamin K just after birth. The injection quickly raises the infant's vitamin K level to normal and maintains the normal level for several months. Infants who do not receive vitamin K prophylaxis at birth will take several weeks (formula fed) to several months (breast fed) to attain normal vitamin K levels. Formula contains higher levels of vitamin K than human milk. VKDB occurs in two forms:

- **Early onset form** occurs within the first 24 hours after birth, and is related to maternal medications that interfere with Vitamin K.
- **Late onset form** occurs after two weeks of age, because of exclusive breastfeeding, diarrhea, hepatitis, cystic fibrosis, alpha 1-antitrypsin disease, or celiac disease.

VACCINES

There are a number of different types of **vaccines**:

- **Conjugated forms:** An organism is altered and then joined (conjugated) with another substance, such as a protein, to potentiate immune response (such as conjugated Hib).
- **Killed virus vaccines:** The virus has been killed but can still cause an immune response (such as inactivated poliovirus).
- **Live virus vaccines:** The virus is live but in a weakened (attenuated) form so that it doesn't cause the disease but confers immunity (such as measles vaccine).
- **Recombinant forms:** The organism is genetically altered and for example, may use proteins rather than the whole cell to stimulate immunity (such as Hepatitis B and acellular pertussis vaccine).
- **Toxoid:** A toxin (antigen) that has been weakened by the use of heat or chemicals so it is too weak to cause disease but stimulates antibodies.

Some vaccines are given shortly after birth; others begin at 2 months, 12 months, or 2 years and some later in childhood.

HEPATITIS B VACCINE

Hepatitis B is transmitted through blood and body fluids, including during birth; therefore, it is now recommended for all newborns as well as all those <18 and those in high risk groups >18 (drug users, men having sex with men, those with multiple sex partners, partners of those with HBV, and healthcare workers). Hepatitis B can cause serious liver disease leading to liver cancer. Three injections of monovalent HepB are required to confer immunity:

- Birth (within 12 hours).
- Between 1-2 months.
- ≥24 weeks.

Note: If combination vaccines are given after the birth dose then a dose at 4 months can be given.

If the mother is Hepatitis B positive, the child should be given both the monovalent HepB vaccination as well as HepB immune globulin within 12 hours of birth. Adverse reactions include local irritation and fever. Severe allergic reactions can occur to those allergic to baker's yeast.

INACTIVATED POLIOVIRUS VACCINE

Poliomyelitis is a serious viral infection that can cause paralysis and death. Prior to introduction of a vaccine in 1955, polio was responsible for >20,000 cases in the United States each year. There

12

have been no cases of polio caused by the poliovirus for >20 years in the United States, but it still occurs in some third world countries, so continuing vaccinations is very important. Oral polio vaccine (OPV) is no longer recommended in the United States because it carries a very slight risk of causing the disease (1:2.4 million). Children require 4 doses of injectable polio vaccine (IPV):

- 2 months
- 4 months
- 6-18 months
- 4-6 years (booster dose)

IPV is contraindicated for those who have had a severe reaction to neomycin, streptomycin, or polymyxin B. Rare allergic reactions can occur, but there are almost no serious problems caused by this vaccine.

DIPHTHERIA, TETANUS, AND PERTUSSIS VACCINE

Diphtheria and pertussis (whooping cough) are highly contagious bacterial diseases of the upper respiratory tract. Cases of diphtheria are now rare however, recent outbreaks of pertussis have occurred in the United States. Tetanus is a bacterial infection contracted through cuts, wounds, and scratches. The **diphtheria, tetanus, and pertussis (DTaP) vaccine** is recommended for all children. DTaP requires 5 doses:

- 2 months
- 4 months
- 6 months
- 5-18 months
- 4-6 years (or at 11-12 years if booster missed between 4-6)

ROTAVIRUS VACCINE

Rotavirus is a cause of significant morbidity and mortality in children, especially in developing countries, but most children, without vaccination, will suffer from severe diarrhea caused by rotavirus within the first 5 years of life. The new rotavirus vaccine is advised for all infants but should not be initiated after 12 weeks or administered after 32 weeks, so there is a narrow window of opportunity. Three doses are required:

- 2 months (between 6-12 weeks)
- 4 months
- 6 months

HEPTAVALENT PNEUMOCOCCAL CONJUGATE VACCINE

Heptavalent pneumococcal conjugate vaccine (PCV-7) (Prevnar®) was released for use in the United States in 2001 for treatment of children under 2 years old. It provides immunity to 7 serotypes of *Streptococcus pneumoniae* to protect against invasive pneumococcal disease, such as pneumonia, otitis media, bacteremia, and meningitis. Because children are most at risk ≤1, vaccinations begin early:

Administration:

- 1st dose: 6-8 weeks.
- 2nd dose: 4 months.

- 3rd dose: 6 months.
- 4th dose: 12-18 months.

HAEMOPHILUS INFLUENZAE TYPE B VACCINE

Haemophilus influenzae **type B (HIB) vaccine** (HibTITER® and PedavaxHIB®) protects against infection with *Haemophilus influenzae,* which can cause serious respiratory infections, pneumonia, meningitis, bacteremia, and pericarditis in children ≤5 years old. *Administration:*

- 1st dose: 2 months.
- 2nd dose: 4 months.
- 3rd dose: 6 months (may be required, depending upon the brand of vaccine).
- Last dose: 12-15 months (this booster dose must be given at least 2 months after the earlier doses for those who start at a later age than 2 months.

ASSESSING COMFORT LEVEL

Unlike older children or adults, neonates can not self-report pain. Several tools have been developed to **standardize the assessment of pain** by utilizing behavioral measures in the term and preterm infant. A particularly useful standard, developed at the University of Toronto, is the **Premature Infant Pain Profile (PIPP).** The PIPP utilizes 7 measurable indicators of pain that are translated into a final score. The neonate is observed before the procedure to obtain baseline data and then for 30 seconds after the procedure. The indicators scored are: Nasolabial furrow; eye squeeze; brow bulge; change in oxygen saturation; change in heart rate; behavioral state; and gestational age. Each of these categories is given a score of 0-3, with higher scores indicating elevated levels of pain. Other tools include the **Neonatal Facial Coding System** and the **Neonatal Infant Pain Profile**.

SUCROSE ANALGESIA

Sucrose analgesia (Sweet-Ease™) is used to relieve stress and discomfort in infants before and during medical procedures, such as heel sticks, IV insertion, injections, suctioning, and insertion of NG tubes. Sweet-Ease™, a commercially prepared product, is 24% sucrose in an oral solution into which a standard pacifier is dipped and given to the infant, usually 2 minutes before a procedure. The pacifier may be re-dipped every 2 minutes for a total of 4 times. If the infant cannot suck, 0.1 mL of solution is placed on the anterior tongue with a medical syringe with the same frequency. For more painful procedures, such as lumbar puncture and circumcision, sucrose analgesia may be used in conjunction with other forms of analgesia to provide comfort. Contraindications include: <32 weeks gestation, hyperglycemia, history of asphyxia or intolerance to feedings, critical illness, paralysis, opioid sedation, and infants NPO for surgery unless cleared by anesthesiologist.

NEONATAL ANALGESICS

ACETAMINOPHEN

Acetaminophen (Tylenol®) is used both for control of mild to moderate pain and fever. Acetaminophen can be administered orally and rectally, but absorption is less reliable with the rectal route. Acetaminophen has a half-life of 4 hours, is conjugated in the liver, and is excreted through the kidneys. **Oral dosage** is typically 24 mg/kg as a loading dose and 12 mg/kg every four hours (or 8 hours in infants <32 weeks); **rectal dosage** is 36 mg/kg (loading), followed by 24 mg/kg every 8 hours. Serum levels should be checked if treatment is to continue for >24 hours. Serum levels of 12 to 24 mg/L are required for adequate pain control. Acetaminophen is commonly used for control of pain after **circumcision**, although it is not sufficient for pain control during the procedure.

FENTANYL AND MORPHINE

Fentanyl and morphine are opioid **analgesics/narcotics** that treat moderate-to-severe pain.

- **Fentanyl** is for painful dressing changes or procedures. Duration of action is 1 to 2 hours and half-life is 2 to 4 hours. Dosage is 1 to 4 µg/kg every 1 to 2 hours or by continuous infusion. Rapid tolerance develops, requiring higher doses to create the same relief, and increasing the chance of overdose. Fentanyl is metabolized by the liver and excreted by the kidneys. Side effects of fentanyl include respiratory depression, peripheral vasodilatation, inhibition of intestinal peristalsis, and chest wall rigidity at higher doses, which compromises ventilation. Fentanyl is less likely to cause hypotension than morphine.
- **Morphine** is for postoperative pain. Duration of action is 3 to 4 hours, and half-life is 2 to 4 hours. Morphine is metabolized by the liver to an inactive metabolite and excreted by the kidneys; 2 to 12% is excreted unchanged in the urine. Dosage is 0.02 to 0.1 mg/kg every 1 to 4 hours or by continuous infusion. Side effects of morphine include respiratory depression, histamine release, and seizures.

NON-PHARMACOLOGIC INTERVENTIONS FOR NEONATAL PAIN

Interventions that may be used to **reduce or relieve neonatal pain** include:

- Grouped procedures to reduce the number of painful events (care clustering).
- Reduced handling prior to procedures.
- Facilitated tucking (hand swaddling) during procedures (extremities flexed and bound close to trunk reduces response to pain in preterm neonates).
- Swaddling after procedures reduces stress.
- Non-nutritive sucking (pacifier) reduces pain response only while sucking. Pacifier dipped in sucrose (0.05 to 2 mL of 12 to 25%) may be more effective than pacifier only.
- Breastfeeding may reduce pain during procedures.
- MedVac (beanbag) "shrink wrap" conforms to neonate's body and stabilizes the child.

Fluid, Electrolytes, and Glucose Homeostasis

BODY FLUID/FLUID BALANCE

Body fluid is primarily intracellular fluid (ICF) or extracellular space (ECF). Infants and children have proportionately more extracellular fluid (ECF) than adults. At birth, more than half of the child's weight is ECF (by 3 years of age, the balance is more like adults):

- ECF: 20-30% (intrastitial fluid, plasma, transcellular fluid).
- ICF: 40-50% (fluid within the cells).

The fluid compartments are separated by semipermeable membranes that allow fluid and solutes (electrolytes and other substances) to move by osmosis. Fluid also moves through diffusion, filtration, and active transport. In fluid volume deficit, fluid is out of balance and ECF is depleted; an overload occurs with increased concentration of sodium and retention of fluid. Signs of fluid deficit include:

- Restless to lethargic.
- Increasing pulse rate, tachycardia.
- Fontanels depressed.
- ↓ urinary output.
- Normal BP progressing hypotension.
- Dry mucous membranes, thirst.
- ↓ in body weight.

TOTAL BODY WATER

Total body water (TBW) content is the percentage of the body composed of water. An extremely premature infant (24 to 26 weeks of gestation) has a TBW content of 90%. The TBW content drops to 75-80% at full term (40 weeks), compared to 60-65% in adults. Because preterm infants have such a high percentage of TBW, any fluid loss can cause severe problems. Physiological diuresis is fluid loss from the extracellular space, and this is the initial type of fluid loss in neonates. Because intracellular space is relatively small in neonates, there is less fluid available to shift into the extracellular space, so the effects of extracellular fluid loss are much more pronounced on infants than adults. Diuresis continues during the first week after birth, so full term infants lose 5-10% of their weight, and premature infants lose 10-15% of their weight. Diuresis diminishes but slowly continues over the first 1 to 2 years of life. The typical toddler has a TBW content of 60%.

SENSIBLE AND INSENSIBLE WATER LOSS

Sensible water losses occur via urination, stool, and gastric drainage, and can be accurately measured. **Insensible water losses** (IWL) occur as water evaporates from the skin (2/3) or the respiratory tract (1/3). IWL cannot be directly measured. Premature neonates have thin skin that allows for increased amounts of evaporative water loss. As the skin matures and the stratum corneum develops (around 31 weeks of gestation) less water is lost through the skin. A full-term neonate will have an IWL of 12/ml/kg/24 hours at 50% humidity. Factors that increase IWL include prematurity, radiant warmers, phototherapy, fever, low humidity, and tachypnea. Infants who are mechanically ventilated should receive humidified oxygen to negate the IWL through their lungs. The nurse must take into account IWL when providing fluids to neonates.

FLUID DEFICIT

Pediatric fluid deficit must also be carefully estimated and managed. Fluid deficit should be replaced over 3 hours with half the first hour and a quarter in the remaining 2 hours. Fluid deficit is calculated by first finding the **maintenance fluid requirement**:

- Maintenance fluid mL X hours NPO = fluid deficit.

Preoperative deficits usually are treated with lactated Ringer's or 1/ normal saline (which may cause hyperchloremic acidosis). Glucose containing fluids may contribute to hyperglycemia.

Fluid replacement must account for both blood loss and third-space loss:

- Blood: Replacement may be with lactated Ringers (3 mL to 1 mL blood loss) or 5% albumin colloid (1 mL to 1 mL blood loss) to maintain hematocrit at predetermined adequate minimal level:
  - Infants and neonates: >30% (may be as high as 40-50%).
  - Older children: 20-26%.

Blood is replaced with packed red blood cells when the allowable blood loss threshold is exceeded. (Continued)

Allowable blood loss is calculated by the following formula based on the infant's average hematocrit:

- .Average hematocrit = (Beginning hematocrit + minimum adequate hematocrit) / 2.
- Allowable blood loss = [Estimated blood loss X (beginning hematocrit – minimum adequate hematocrit)] / average hematocrit.

Blood loss should be monitored carefully to determine when it exceeds the allowable blood loss. **Volume of packed red blood cell replacement** is based on the hematocrit of packed cells, 75%:

- Packed red blood cells in mL = [Estimated blood loss – allowable blood loss) X minimum adequate hematocrit] / packed red blood cell hematocrit of 75.

If blood loss is in excess of 1-2 blood volumes, then 10-15 mL/kg of platelets and FFP are administered. **Third space loss** after surgery can only be estimated based on the degree of trauma:

- Minor: 3-4 mL/kg/hr; Moderate: 5-6 mL/kg/hr; Severe: 7-10 mL/kg/hr.

Lactated Ringers is most commonly used to replace third space loss.

SODIUM, HYPONATREMIA, AND HYPERNATREMIA

Sodium (Na) regulates fluid volume, osmolality, acid-base balance, and activity in the muscles, nerves and myocardium. It is the primary cation (positive ion) in ECF, necessary to maintain ECF levels needed for tissue perfusion:

- Normal neonatal value: 133-146 mEq/L.
- Hyponatremia: <133 mEq/L. (Critical value <120).
- Hypernatremia: >146 mEq/L. (Critical value >160).

Hyponatremia develops with excessive water gain or excessive sodium loss. Late symptoms include apnea, irritability, twitching, and seizures when serum sodium drops below 120 mEq/L, but infants are often asymptomatic. In the first days after birth, hyponatremia is usually secondary to excessive water gain (dilutional hyponatremia), reflected in a weight gain or absence of expected weight loss. Conditions causing dilutional hyponatremia include syndrome of inappropriate antidiuretic hormone (SIADH), renal dysfunction with decreased urine output, and overhydration. Treatment involves identifying and treating underlying cause, restricting fluid, and replacing sodium if necessary. **Hypernatremia** is caused by dehydration, excess use of sodium containing solutions, and diabetes insipidus. Late symptoms include seizures. Underlying cause must be identified and treated.

HYPOCALCEMIA

The ionized form of **serum calcium** is the only biologically available form in the body.

- Cord: 8.2 to 11.2 mg/dL
- 0 to 10 days: 7.6 to 10.4 mg/dL
- 11 days to 1 yr: 9.0 to 11.0 mg/dL
- Critical value for hypocalcemia: <7 mg/dL

Signs of **hypocalcemia** include jitteriness, irritability, stridor, tetany, high-pitched cry, seizures, and decreased myocardial contractility, with decreased cardiac output. An electrocardiogram may show a prolonged QT interval and a flattened T-wave. Early onset hypocalcemia usually presents in the first 3 days of life and is associated with prematurity, birth asphyxia, and infants of diabetic mothers. Late onset hypocalcemia presents after the first week of life and is associated with DiGeorge syndrome, hyperphosphatemia, vitamin D deficiency, magnesium deficiency, diuretic therapy, and hypoparathyroidism. Hypocalcemia is treated with a slow infusion of calcium gluconate. Rapid infusion may cause bradycardia. Tissue infiltration with calcium causes necrosis, so the administration site must be monitored.

HYPERCALCEMIA

Hypercalcemia (>12 mg/dL) is rare, occurring less often than hypocalcemia. Signs of hypercalcemia include: Vomiting; constipation; hypertension; hypotonia; lethargy and seizures. Possible causes of hypercalcemia include: Congenital hyperparathyroidism; maternal hypoparathyroidism; hypervitaminosis D; hyperthyroidism; hypophosphatasia; subcutaneous fat necrosis; Williams syndrome; and adrenal insufficiency. Idiopathic hypercalcemia is diagnosed when no other cause can be found. Iatrogenic hypercalcemia occurs because of excess administration of calcium or vitamin D, or phosphate deprivation. Treatment depends on the exact cause, but may include:

- Correction of the underlying cause.
- Furosemide (Lasix) after adequate hydration to increase calcium excretion.
- Glucocorticoids to inhibit intestinal absorption of calcium.
- Use of low calcium and low vitamin D formulas.

MAGNESIUM, HYPERMAGNESEMIA, AND HYPOMAGNESEMIA

Magnesium is the second most abundant intercellular cation:

- Neonate: 1.5-2.2 mg/dL.
- Critical values: <1.2 mg/dL and >3 mg/dL (neonates)

Hypermagnesemia most commonly results from maternal administration of magnesium prior to delivery. Maternal serum chemistries are reflected in newborn blood values. Magnesium is used in

18

the pregnant woman as a tocolytic agent to stop pre-term labor, and also for treatment of pre-eclampsia. Signs of hypermagnesemia in an infant include hypotonia, hyporeflexia, constipation, low blood pressure, apnea, and marked flushing secondary to vasodilatation. Elevated magnesium blocks neurosynaptic transmission by interfering with the release of acetylcholine. Treatment is usually supportive, as the elevated serum magnesium will be cleared by the infant's kidneys. In severe cases the infant may require respiratory and/or blood pressure support.

Hypomagnesemia in neonates occurs with preterm birth, respiratory distress syndrome, and neonatal hepatitis. *Symptoms* include:

- Neuromuscular excitability/ tetany.
- Seizure and coma.
- Tachycardia with ventricular arrhythmias.
- Respiratory depression.

Treatment includes diagnosing underlying cause and magnesium replacement.

SERUM POTASSIUM CHANGES AFTER BIRTH

Electrolyte levels in the newborn reflect those of the mother at birth. Shortly after birth, within the first 24 to 72 hours, **serum potassium** concentrations are expected to rise without exogenous potassium delivery and with normal renal function, resulting from a shift of potassium from the intracellular space to the extracellular space. **Potassium shift** is more extreme in premature infants and can result in life- threatening hyperkalemia. Over the next several days, the potassium level will fall to normal in an infant with normally functioning kidneys. Preterm infants' serum electrolytes, including potassium, should be carefully monitored in the first 48 hours of life and until values have stabilized.

- Normal neonatal values: 3.7 to 5.9 mEq/L
- Hyperkalemia: >6 mEq/L; critical value: >6.5 mEq/L
- Hypokalemia: <3.5 mEq/L; critical value: <2.5 mEq/L

HYPERKALEMIA

Hyperkalemia is a serum potassium level greater than 6 mEq/L in a non-hemolyzed blood sample. Squeezing the infant's heel too hard during blood collection can cause the sample to hemolyze and give an artificially elevated laboratory value. Causes of hyperkalemia in the newborn fall into 3 categories:

- Excessive potassium supplementation.
- Transcellular shift, where potassium concentrated inside cells moves outside cells, due to low pH, cellular damage, intraventricular hemorrhage or trauma.
- Decreased potassium secretion by the kidneys, due to congenital adrenal hyperplasia with elevated secretion of aldosterone or renal failure.

Cardiac manifestations of hyperkalemia include potentially fatal arrhythmias like bradycardia, tachycardia, supraventricular fibrillation, and ventricular fibrillation. EKG shows peaked T waves (earliest sign), and a widened QRS complex.

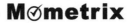

TREATMENT

Hyperkalemia must be treated promptly because it may develop into a lethal cardiac arrhythmia, especially if the blood potassium value is >7 mEq/L and the infant's electrocardiogram shows abnormalities. Follow these steps to lower potassium levels:

- Discontinue all potassium administration.
- Elevate the blood pH by inducing hyperventilation.
- Give sodium bicarbonate to shift extracellular potassium back inside cells.
- Administer insulin and/or inhaled albuterol to enhance the shift of extracellular potassium back inside cells. *Monitor glucose levels closely.*
- Increase excretion of potassium by giving furosemide (Lasix) or sodium polystyrene sulfonate (Kayexalate).
- Give calcium gluconate concurrently to help stabilize the myocardium and lessen the chance of the infant developing an arrhythmia.
- In extreme cases, consider dialysis or exchange transfusion.

HYPOKALEMIA

Hypokalemia is a serum potassium level less than 3.5 mEq/L. Common causes of hypokalemia are chronic diuretic use and excessive nasogastric drainage. Alkalosis accentuates hypokalemia by triggering the sequestration of potassium from the extracellular fluid to inside the cell. Electrocardiograph manifestations of hypokalemia include a flattened T wave (earliest manifestation), ST segment depression, and appearance of U waves (second recovery wave following the T wave). These changes are identical to those seen with hypomagnesemia. Hypokalemia is usually not of concern until the level drops below 3.0 mEq/L. Signs of hypokalemia include cardiac arrhythmias, ileus, and lethargy. *Treatment* is with Slow-K and can be intravenous or oral. Rapid administration of potassium is associated with possible life-threatening cardiac dysfunction.

PARENTERAL INFUSION

Most infants in the NICU require intravenous fluids, and there are a number of different types of access for **parenteral infusions**:

- **Umbilical cord catheterization (arterial, venous)**: This is limited to a few days only.
- **PICC line:** This allows for long-term use without repeated IV insertions. It is particularly useful for ELBW babies although they pose the danger of thrombosis, infection, and infiltration. Percutaneous insertion sites include the saphenous, antecubital, axillary, basilic, cephalic, and external jugular veins.
- **Peripheral venous access:** This is used for short-term access. Extremely small catheters and introducers (Quick-cath®) may extend use to 5-7 days. There is increased risk of infiltration and skin necrosis, especially in the foot.

The catheter or needle should be secured, but must allow visualization and the site should be checked at least every hour during administration of fluids.

TOTAL PARENTERAL NUTRITION

A preterm or compromised infant may not tolerate enteral feedings for several weeks, so the infant's nutritional needs are met with IV **total parenteral nutrition** (TPN). The goals of TPN are to:

- Provide normal metabolism.
- Support growth without significant morbidity.
- Prevent essential fatty acid deficiency.
- Balance nitrogen.
- Prevent muscle wasting (catabolism).

TPN is started after birth. Dextrose provides the majority of calories, but to avoid elevated blood glucose levels, dextrose is administered at 6mg/kg/min and increased to 10 to 12 mg/kg/min over several days. The infant's serum glucose is monitored regularly for hyperglycemia. Protein content is slowly increased over several days to 3 to 3.5 g/kg/day. Lipids, required for calories and the absorption of fat-soluble vitamins like A, D, and E, are started at 0.5/gm/kg/day and increased to 3 to 3.5 gm/kg/day. Other components of TPN include sodium, potassium, calcium, phosphorus, magnesium, trace elements, and vitamins. TPN may be administered through a peripheral IV line for <one week and a central line for longer periods.

INTRAVENOUS LIPIDS

Intravenous lipids are an important component of total parenteral nutrition (TPN) because they provide essential fatty acids, a concentrated calorie source (9 calories per gram of fat), and improve delivery of fat-soluble vitamins to infants who cannot tolerate enteral feeds. General guidelines for the administration of IV lipids are to start with 0.5/g/kg on the third day of life and advance slowly to a final administration rate of 3 to 3.5/g/kg/day by 7 to 10 days. Delivery of IV lipids should be continuous over 18 to 24 hours each day. Serum lipid levels should be monitored for hyperlipidemia. Potential *complications* include:

- Risk of kernicterus in infants with elevated unconjugated bilirubin. Free fatty acids displace bilirubin from albumin binding sites. Infusion of lipids should be at the lower level in infants with elevated unconjugated bilirubin.
- Exacerbation of chronic lung disease.
- Exacerbation of persistent pulmonary hypertension.

COMPLICATIONS

Complications of total parenteral nutrition (TPN) result from the presence of the intravenous access (usually a central line) and the development of cholestasis. Both of these events are more common in infants receiving TPN longer than 2 to 3 weeks. The longer an infant receives TPN, the more likely complications will occur. Consequences of prolonged venous access include sepsis, thrombophlebitis, and extravasation of fluid into soft tissue with possible tissue necrosis. Premature infants have an immature hepatobiliary system. One hypothesis for the development of cholestasis is that a lack of fat in the duodenum leads to biliary stasis. Infants requiring TPN are often very ill, may have episodes of shock, or require surgical interventions, all of which contribute to the development of TPN-associated cholestasis. Jaundiced infants show an elevated direct bilirubin in blood serum. Treatment usually involves the discontinuation of TPN, along with the slow introduction of enteral feeds (if possible).

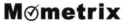

Diagnostic Techniques and Equipment
Umbilical Artery Catheter

Umbilical catheters may be arterial or venous, depending on primary need:

- Arterial: ABG monitoring, continuous arterial BP monitoring, infusion of parenteral fluids.

Umbilical artery catheter placement: A sterile field must be maintained, so the infant's arms and legs are restrained to prevent contamination. The infant's temperature must be monitored and maintained at 36-37 °C (by placing on radiant heater or in heated incubator). The child is placed in supine position and the umbilical cord and surrounding skin cleansed with povidone iodine and then alcohol or sterile water. For infants <1250 g a 3.5 Fr. catheter is used, and for those >1250 g, 5 Fr. catheter. After sterile draping, iris forceps are used to dilate one of the arteries and the catheter inserted. If resistance is felt at the umbilical cord tie, it may need to be loosened. The inserted length correlates to the infant's length (using chart), traveling inferiorly and then superiorly (leg loop). Blood should be aspirated and extremities observed for circulatory compromise. Radiograph verifies correct placement.

Umbilical Vein Catheter

Umbilical catheters may be inserted into the umbilical vein. This is easy to identify as there is only one, it is larger than the arteries, and it is usually open and does not require dilation. Indications for using the umbilical vein include:

- Venous: Exchange transfusions, CVP monitoring, and emergency administration of fluids.

Umbilical vein catheter placement: Catheter size is 3.5 Fr. for ELBW infants or 5 Fr. (most common). Length of placement is estimated by measuring the length from the umbilicus to the sternal notch and multiplying this number by 0.6. The procedure for insertion is similar to that for the umbilical artery, but insertion is usually easier. The catheter should be in the inferior vena cava, above the diaphragm but below right atrium. Placement should be verified by echocardiography, as radiograph may not provide adequate visualization.

PICC Lines

Percutaneously inserted central catheters (PICC) are used for extended intravenous access or those with limited access, and as a transition from umbilical catheters. Insertion sites include the scalp, axilla, and brachial cephalic saphenous veins. The catheter insertion length is measured:

- **Hand/arm:** Insertion site to axilla and to 1 cm above nipple line.
- **Scalp:** Insertion site to 1 cm above nipple line.
- **Leg:** Insertion site to 1 cm above umbilicus.

Topical (EMLA) or local anesthetic is used and the infant's temperature maintained at 36-37 °C. Limbs are restrained to prevent contamination of sterile field. If catheter is inserted in the hand or arm, the infant's head is turned toward insertion site to partially occlude the jugular vein and reduce risk of catheter entering the jugular. After insertion above the waist, the catheter should be in the superior vena cava above the right atrium. PICC lines in lower extremities should lie in the inferior vena cava below the right atrium. AP and lateral radiographs, ultrasound, or echocardiogram verify correct placement.

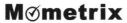

Oxygenation, Non-Invasive Ventilation, and Acid-Base Balance

OXYHEMOGLOBIN DISSOCIATION CURVE

The **oxyhemoglobin dissociation curve** is a graph that plots the percentage of hemoglobin saturated with oxygen (Y-axis) and different partial pressures of oxygen (pO_2 levels) (X-axis.) The neonate has about 70-90% fetal hemoglobin, which carries less oxygen but has a higher affinity for oxygen and greater oxygen saturation than adult hemoglobin, so the curve is different. A curve shift to the right represents conditions where hemoglobin has less affinity for oxygen (greater amounts of oxygen are released). A shift to the left has the opposite implications. Low pH shifts the curve to the right, enabling increased off-loading of hemoglobin to tissues. Elevated oxygen shifts the curve to the left, causing increased affinity of hemoglobin for oxygen in the lungs. Small changes in fetal PO_2 result in greater loading or unloading of oxygen compared to adult hemoglobin. Because of the increased affinity for oxygen, lower tissue oxygen levels are needed to trigger the unload of oxygen. Thus, the infant will have a lower PO_2 and oxygen saturation before cyanosis is evident.

NON-INVASIVE MONITORING OF INFANT ON OXYGEN

Non-invasive monitoring of the neonate receiving **oxygen** includes:

- **Heart rate monitor**: Should show beats per minute as well as a visual depiction of the heart rhythm.
- **Respiratory monitor**: Should show respiratory rate as well as a visual wave showing the pattern of breathing. Alarms should be turned on for apnea and tachypnea.
- **Blood pressure monitor**: Peripheral cuff type monitoring, this does not need to be continuous but needs to be done at regular intervals determined by the physician or practitioner.
- **Pulse oximetry:** Should be a continuous monitoring with alarms set for ordered lower limits.
- **Oxygen analyzer:** Shows the oxygen level being delivered to the neonate.

NON-INVASIVE TRANSCUTANEOUS O₂/CO₂ MONITORING

Non-invasive **transcutaneous O_2/CO_2 monitoring** includes skin oxygen tension ($TCPO_2$) and carbon dioxide tension ($TCPCO_2$). One or two leads are placed on the infant's skin over any part of the body that allows good contact. O_2 and CO_2 diffuse through the skin and monitors provide a digital display. If right-to-left shunting is suspected, then leads are usually placed on right shoulder and lower abdomen or leg (above and below the ductus arteriosus). The electrodes are calibrated (usually every 4 hours to ensure accuracy), and then heat (43-44 °C) the underlying skin, but they must be left in place for 15-minutes after calibration to ensure adequate heating of the skin. The electrodes can cause erythema (first-degree burns), so they should be repositioned every 2-4 hours. The electrodes should not be placed beneath the infant because the pressure against it can impede circulation.

END-TIDAL CO₂ MONITORS

End-tidal CO_2 monitors are used to confirm correct placement of endotracheal tubes during intubation and to ensure adequate oxygenation. Both sidestream analysis with a double lumen ETT and mainstream analysis within the ventilator circuit are used. Clinical assessment alone is not adequate:

- **Capnography** is attached to the ETT and provides a waveform graph, showing the varying concentrations of CO_2 in real time throughout each ventilation (with increased CO_2 on expiration) and can indicate changes in respiratory status.

23

A typical waveform rises with expiration (indicating CO_2 level), plateaus, and then falls with inspiration (and intake of oxygen). Changes in the height or shape of the waveform can indicate respiratory compromise. Pressure of end-tidal CO_2 ($PETCO_2$) is useful for neonates with normal lung function or in premature infants with mild-moderate lung disease, but results may be inaccurate if there is a large alveolar-arterial gradient.

NEONATAL PULSE OXIMETRY

Pulse oximetry is a means of monitoring the saturation level of the **hemoglobin** in the blood. For example, a reading of 98% indicates that 98% of the hemoglobin available is bound to oxygen or saturated with oxygen. A machine uses infrared light to read the hemoglobin. Several things can affect the accuracy of this reading.

- The **perfusion status** of the neonate. If the infant is suffering from a condition that results in poor perfusion (hypovolemia, hypotension, etc.), the pulse oximetry reading will be inaccurate, as the machine will have difficulty reading the blood.
- **Phototherapy** used for jaundice will also cause inaccurate readings, because like the tool used in pulse oximetry, it is a light.
- Use of **dopamine**, a potent vasoconstricting drug that causes problems reading the blood for oxygen levels if the veins are constricted, affecting blood flow.

Pulse oximetry is now a recommended screening tool for congenital heart defects. While not diagnostic, it provides information that can either rule out congenital heart defects, or trigger further investigation.

NEONATAL OXYGEN ADMINISTRATION

Principles of **neonatal oxygen administration**:

- Oxygen administration should be titrated to the need of the particular infant. The determining factor to titrate to should be PO_2 levels as measured from arterial blood. Oxygen concentration should be titrated to keep the arterial PO_2 level between 50 and 80 mmHg.
- Supplemental oxygen concentration should be initiated at 21% (30% in preterm infants) and then titrated up to prevent injuries from excessive oxygenation.
- Oxygen should never be given without some method of monitoring the level of oxygen in the infant's blood at all times, such as with pulse oximetry or arterial blood gas studies.
- Oxygen given to a neonate should always be humidified at 30-40%. Oxygen administered without humidification dries the nasal passages, increasing respiratory distress.
- Oxygen should also be warmed to 31-34 °C. Failing to warm the oxygen can cause cold stress for the infant.
- Any adjustments to the concentration of oxygen must be done slowly because an abrupt change can cause sudden vasoconstriction.

FLOW-INFLATING BAG AND MASK VENTILATION

Bag and mask ventilation is indicated for persistent apnea or gasping respirations, bradycardia (<100 bpm), and persistent cyanosis unrelieved by free-flowing oxygen.

Flow-inflating bag and mask (connected to oxygen flow, which inflates bag) equipment includes:

- Oxygen inlet.
- Flow control valve.
- Pressure manometer attachment.
- Patient outlet for mask attachment.

Advantages: Flow-inflating bag and mask ventilation has the ability to deliver anywhere from 21% (room air) to 100% oxygen; any pressure desired can be set. This type of bag and mask also has the ability to maintain positive end-expiratory pressure (PEEP) and CPAP.

Disadvantages: Because this bag must be connected to a gas (oxygen) source to inflate, it can only be used where a gas supply exists. It requires some experience to deliver the desired quantity of air with each breath. The high pressures possible with this type of equipment make over-inflation of the lungs possible, resulting in pneumothorax. A complete seal is necessary to deliver a tidal volume.

SELF-INFLATING BAG AND MASK VENTILATION

Self-inflating bag and mask (does not require gas source) equipment includes:

- Air inlet.
- Oxygen inlet.
- Patient outlet for mask attachment.
- Valve assembly.
- Oxygen reservoir.
- Pop-off valve.
- Pressure manometer attachment.

Advantages: Self-inflating bag and mask ventilation is simple to use and does not require much practice or experience to operate. It can be operated anywhere even if no oxygen source is near and can easily deliver a tidal volume.

Disadvantages: These bags usually have a pop-off valve that will open at a pressure set by the manufacturer to prevent over inflation of the lungs. This valve popping off can prevent the ability to deliver enough pressure to ventilate very noncompliant lungs. Another disadvantage is that if 90% or higher oxygen delivery is desired, this equipment must have a reservoir attached to deliver this concentration. The inability to deliver PEEP is also a disadvantage to the self-inflating bag and mask.

NON-INVASIVE POSITIVE PRESSURE VENTILATORS

Non-invasive positive pressure ventilators provide air through a tight-fitting nasal or facemask, usually pressure cycled, avoiding the need for intubation and reducing the danger of hospital-acquired infection and mortality rates. It can be used for acute respiratory failure and pulmonary edema. There are 2 types of non-invasive positive pressure ventilators:

- **CPAP** (Continuous positive airway pressure) provides a steady stream of pressurized air throughout both inspiration and expiration. CPAP improves breathing by decreasing preload and afterload for patients with congestive heart failure. It reduces the effort required for breathing and improves compliance of the lung.

- **Bi-PAP** (Bi-level positive airway pressure) provides a steady stream of pressurized air as CPAP, but it senses inspiratory effort and increases pressure during inspiration only. Bi-PAP pressures for inspiration and expiration can be set independently. Machines can be programmed with a backup rate to ensure a set number of respirations per minute.

POSITIVE PRESSURE VENTILATORS

Positive pressure ventilators assist respiration by applying pressure directly to the airway, inflating the lungs, forcing expansion of the alveoli, and facilitating gas exchange. Generally, endotracheal intubation or tracheostomy is necessary to maintain positive pressure ventilation. There are 3 basic kinds of positive pressure ventilators:

- **Pressure cycled:** This type of ventilation is usually used for short-term treatment in adolescents or adults. The IPPB machine is the most common type. This delivers a flow of air to a preset pressure and then cycles off. Airway resistance or changes in compliance can affect volume of air and may compromise ventilation.
- **Time cycled:** This type of ventilation regulates the volume of air the infant receives by controlling the length of inspiration and the flow rate. This type of ventilator is used almost exclusively for neonates and infants.
- **Volume cycled:** This type of ventilation provides a preset flow of pressurized air during inspiration and then cycles off and allows passive expiration, providing a fairly consistent volume of air.

OXYGEN HOOD

Oxygen can be delivered through a clear **oxygen hood** (usually made of plastic) fitted over the infant's head. This type of delivery is appropriate for an infant who has a mild form of RDS and can maintain normal carbon dioxide levels in his blood, only needing supplemental oxygen. A blender that mixes the oxygen with water, thus humidifying it is usually used with a hood. When the hood is being used for oxygen delivery, it is important that it fit the infant correctly. A hood too large will allow oxygen to escape and lower the concentration the infant is receiving, a hood too small will irritate the infant's skin at contact points. If the infant is to be held for feedings or otherwise removed from the hood, a secondary delivery tool should be available.

NASAL CANNULA DELIVERY OF OXYGEN

A **nasal cannula** is used for the delivery of a neonate who has a long term need for oxygen and is starting to develop motor skills needing the mobility that a cannula allows. The cannula should be the correct size for the infant. The application of a cannula involves putting some kind of skin protection on the infant's cheeks, such as a piece of OpSite® or some other kind of barrier. The tubing is then taped to this barrier to avoid skin irritation. The nares should be frequently assessed for patency. Infants are obligatory nose breathers (they must breathe through their nose) and if mucous or formula plugs the holes in the cannula, they will not be getting the concentration of oxygen they need. Suction the nares as often as needed to keep them clear.

HIGH FREQUENCY JET VENTILATION

High frequency jet ventilation (HFJV) (Life Pulse®) directs a high velocity stream of air into the lungs in a long spiraling spike that forces carbon dioxide against the walls, penetrating dead space and providing gas exchange by using small tidal volumes of 1-3 mL/kg, much smaller than with conventional mechanical ventilation. Because the jet stream technology is effective for short distances, the valve and pressure transducer must be placed by the infant's head. Inhalation is controlled while expiration is passive, but the rate of respiration is up to 11 per second ("panting" respirations). HFJV may be used in conjunction with low-pressure conventional ventilation to increase flow to alveoli. HFJV reduces barotrauma because of the low tidal volume and low pressure. HFJV is used for numerous conditions, including evolving chronic lung disease, pulmonary interstitial emphysema, bronchopulmonary dysplasia, and hypoxemic respiratory failure. It reduces mean airway pressure (MAP) and the oxygenation index. Treatment with HFJV may reduce the need for ECMO.

HIGH FREQUENCY OSCILLATORY VENTILATION

High frequency oscillatory ventilation provides pressurized ventilation with tidal volumes approximately equal to dead space at about 150 breaths per minutes (bpm). Pressure is usually higher with HFOV than HFJV in order to maintain expansion of the alveoli and to keep the airway open during gas exchange. Oxygenation is regulated separately. HFOV has both an active inspiration and expiration, so the respiratory cycle is completely controlled. HFOV reduces pulmonary vascular resistance and improves ventilation-perfusion matching and oxygenation without injuring the lung, reducing the risk of barotrauma. HFOV is used for respiratory distress syndrome, persistent pulmonary hypertension of the newborn (PPHN) associated with meconium aspiration syndrome (MAS). Other indications are air leak syndromes, pulmonary interstitial emphysema, and congenital diaphragmatic hernia. Infants in respiratory distress may be placed on HFOV immediately after birth instead of on conventional ventilation to avoid pulmonary damage.

ENDOTRACHEAL INTUBATION

The difficult airway of neonates makes choosing an age-appropriate **endotracheal tube** (ETT) very important. The formula for estimating ETT sizes:

$$[Age (yr) + 16] / 4 = ETT \text{ size (internal diameter in mm)}$$

Usually the depth an ETT can be inserted is estimated at 3 times the internal diameter of the ETT (or 12 + age / 2 = length). An acceptable ETT leak is 15-20 cm H_2O pressure. The ETT may be inserted nasally or orally. Premedication (morphine or fentanyl and midazolam) is used to relieve stress on the neonate. Atropine may be given to block vagal response. ETT placement should immediately be verified by auscultation and radiograph, ultrasound, or disposable end-tidal carbon dioxide detectors may be used. Esophageal intubation is indicated if no air exchange is detected bilaterally or if there is air sound over left upper abdomen. The tube may be too high if air sounds are diminished and too low if the right lung is better ventilated than the left.

VENTILATOR MANAGEMENT

There are many types of ventilators now in use, and the specific directions for use of each type must be followed carefully, but there are general principles that apply to all **ventilator management.** The following should be monitored:

- **Type of ventilation:** volume-cycled, pressure-cycled, negative-pressure, HFJV, HFOV, CPAP, Bi-PAP.
- **Control mode:** controlled ventilation, assisted ventilation, synchronized intermittent mandatory [allows spontaneous breaths between ventilator controlled inhalation/exhalation], positive-end expiratory pressure (PEEP) [positive pressure at end of expiration], CPAP, Bi-PAP.
- **Tidal volume** (T_v) range should be set in relation to respiratory rate.
- **Inspiratory-expiratory ratio** $(I: E)$ usually ranges from 1:2-1:5, but may vary.
- **Respiratory rate** will depend upon T_v and $PaCO_2$ target.
- **Fraction of inspired oxygen** (FiO_2) [percentage of oxygen in the inspired air], usually ranging from 21-100%, usually maintained <40% to avoid toxicity.

27

- **Sensitivity** determines the effort needed to trigger inspiration.
- **Pressure** controls the pressure exerted in delivering T_v.
- **Rate of flow** controls the L/min speed of T_v.

VILI

Ventilation-induced lung injury (VILI) is damage caused by mechanical ventilation. It is common in acute distress syndrome (ARDS) but can affect any ventilation patient. VILI comprises 4 interrelated elements:

- **Barotrauma**: Damage to the lung caused by excessive pressure.
- **Volutrauma**: Alveolar damage related to high tidal volume ventilation.
- **Atelectotrauma**: Injury caused by repetitive forced opening and closing of alveoli.
- **Biotrauma**: Inflammatory response.

In VILI, essentially the increased pressure and tidal volume over-distends the alveoli, which rupture, and air moves into the interstitial tissue resulting in pulmonary interstitial emphysema. With continued ventilation, the air in the interstitium moves into the subcutaneous tissue and may result in pneumopericardium and pneumomediastinum, or rupture the pleural sac can cause tension pneumothorax and mediastinal shift, which can cause respiratory failure and cardiac arrest. VILI has caused a change in ventilation procedures with lower tidal volumes and pressures used as well as newer forms of ventilation, HFJV and HFOV, preferred to mechanical ventilation for many patients.

RISK FACTORS WITH ADMINISTRATION OF OXYGEN/VENTILATION

There are **risk factors** associated with administration of oxygen/ventilation:

- High oxygen concentration can result in retinopathy of prematurity (ROP) and blindness.
- The mechanical ventilation used to treat a neonate's respiratory disease exerts pressure on the vascular system feeding the lungs; this includes pressure on the pulmonary artery, which comes out of the heart. If this pressure on the pulmonary artery is great enough, cardiac output can be lessened. Lowering the positive pressure settings on the ventilator can alleviate some of this pressure, thus improving cardiac output. Cardiac output can also be supplemented by giving the infant an infusion of extra fluid. This helps to raise cardiac output by enough to compensate for the increased pressure from the ventilator pressures that the heart must overcome to keep the body well oxygenated.
- Oxygenation during resuscitation has been recommended to start at 21% (up to 30% in a preterm newborn) to prevent injuries that can occur from hyperoxygenation. During CPR, oxygen should be administered at 100%.

CHEST TUBE INSERTION/REMOVAL FOR PNEUMOTHORAX

Chest tubes are inserted in the neonate to treat pneumothorax causing cardiac or respiratory compromise or pleural effusion. **Transillumination** may be used to identify the area of pneumothorax but a **chest x-ray** is more accurate. An 8 to 12 Fr. chest tube is placed anteriorly for collections of air and posteriorly/laterally for fluid. The infant is supine with the arm at 90° on the insertion side. The insertion sites are

- **Anterior**: midclavicular line, second or third intercostal space.
- **Posterior/lateral**: anterior axillary line, fourth, fifth, or sixth intercostal space.

Lidocaine is instilled and an incision made over the rib below the target intercostal space. The tissue is spread and the pleura punctured above the rib with a hemostat, expelling air. The chest tube is inserted 2 to 3 cm in preterm and 3 to 4 cm in full-term infants. The purse-string suture is tightened and the chest tube attached to 2 or 3 bottles or a self-contained Pleur-evac® underwater seal system. An x-ray is taken to confirm placement. The chest tube is removed quickly and pressure dressing applied if there is no bubbling for 24 hours and radiograph is clear.

PLEUR-EVAC SYSTEM

A chest tube is attached to a three-chamber system called a **Pleur-Evac.** As the name indicates, there are three separate chambers in this collection system:

- The first chamber is the **collection chamber**. This chamber is where the air and/or fluid that is being drained from the pleural space as a result of a pulmonary air leak. Bubbling in this chamber is the result of air being pumped out of the pleural space and is expected.
- The second chamber is the **water seal chamber**; this chamber is where the water in an amount prescribed by the physician is placed to create the vacuum necessary to pull the fluid and/or air out of the pleural space. The amount of water placed in this chamber affects the amount of pressure and should be carefully monitored to make sure it remains at the ordered level. Bubbling in this chamber indicates a leak and must be investigated.
- The third chamber is the **suction chamber**, which is responsible for the suction that creates the pressure removing the air from the pleural space.

NEEDLE ASPIRATION FOR PNEUMOTHORAX

Neonates receiving bag and mask ventilation or mechanical ventilation risk developing a **pneumothorax**. Signs of pneumothorax include rapid deterioration, poor oxygenation, tachypnea, increased work breathing, impaired circulation, unequal air entry into lungs, displaced apical heartbeat, and increased transillumination on the affected side. If the neonate's clinical status allows it, a chest x-ray will confirm the diagnosis. Air is removed by **needle aspiration.**

The **equipment** for needle aspiration:

- Oral sucrose
- 1% lidocaine
- Fentanyl
- 21-gauge butterfly needle
- 10 mL syringe
- 3-way stopcock attached to the syringe
- 70% isopropyl alcohol swab
- Sterile gloves

The **procedure** for needle aspiration is as follows:

1. Give oral sucrose.
2. Place infant in supine position.
3. Swab second and third intercostal spaces in midclavicular line with alcohol.
4. Infiltrate site with 1% lidocaine 0.5 mL to 1 mL.
5. Drape insertion site.
6. Give 250 mcg fentanyl over 2 to 3 minutes IV.
7. Insert needle directly into second or third intercostal space in mid-clavicular line until air is aspirated into syringe.
8. Expel air through stopcock.

CARDIOPULMONARY MONITORING

Cardiopulmonary monitoring includes electrocardiogram (ECG) and respiratory sensors. Usually 3 chest ECG leads that record the electrical activity of the heart and sense respiratory movement are placed, and the patterns are recorded on a visual screen. Many computerized monitors have memory capability so that data can be analyzed out of real time. They can also be set to record certain events, such as periods of apnea. Alarm thresholds are set, so that an alarm indicates dangerous changes. Apnea alarms should be both visual and auditory. False alarms may occur and should be thoroughly evaluated for cause, such as loose leads or movement. Home monitors include records of compliance so that a review of data shows the time the monitor was actually in use. Home monitors are used for infants at risk for SIDS. Because of interference problems that might provide inaccurate readings, monitors should never be used as a sole evaluation of cardiopulmonary status. Observation and examination must be used to verify the infant's condition.

INVASIVE BLOOD GAS MONITORING

Invasive blood gas monitoring options include the following:

- **Arterial blood gas (ABG)** is the most informative measurement of blood gas status. If an infant has an umbilical artery catheter, it is easily obtained by aspirating 1-2 mL of blood.
- **Venous blood gas (VBG)** is easier to obtain if an arterial catheter is not in place. In order to compare the values in the VBG with an ABG, make the following calculations:
  - Add 0.05 to the pH of the VBG.
  - Subtract 5-10 mmHg from the PCO_2 of the VBG.
- **Capillary Blood Gas (CBG)** can be obtained with a heel stick, without a venous or arterial line, but the values obtained in a CBG are the least accurate and are rarely useful. The oxygen status of the neonate (reflected in the PO_2) can be estimated by clinical evaluation of the neonate and a noninvasive pulse oximeter reading.

METABOLIC AND RESPIRATORY ACIDOSIS

PATHOPHYSIOLOGY
- Metabolic acidosis
  - Increase in fixed acid and inability to excrete acid, or loss of base, with compensatory increase of CO_2 excretion by lungs.
- Respiratory acidosis
  - Hypoventilation and CO_2 retention, with renal compensatory retention of bicarbonate (HCO_3) and increased excretion of hydrogen.

LABORATORY

- Metabolic acidosis
  - Decreased serum pH and PCO_2 normal if uncompensated and decreased if compensated.
  - Decreased HCO_3.
  - Urine pH <6 if compensated.
- Respiratory acidosis
  - Increased serum pH and increased PCO_2.
  - Increased HCO_3 if compensated and normal if uncompensated.
  - Urine pH >6 if compensated.

CAUSES

- Metabolic acidosis
  - DKA, lactic acidosis, diarrhea, starvation, renal failure, shock, renal tubular acidosis, starvation.
- Respiratory acidosis
  - COPD, overdose of sedative or barbiturate, obesity, severe pneumonia/atelectasis, muscle weakness (Guillain-Barré), mechanical hypoventilation

SYMPTOMS

- Metabolic acidosis
  - Neuro/muscular: drowsiness, confusion, headache, coma
  - Cardiac: decreased BP, arrhythmias, flushed skin
  - GI: nausea, vomiting, abdominal pain, diarrhea
  - Respiratory: deep inspired tachypnea
- Respiratory acidosis
  - Neuro/muscular: drowsiness, dizziness, headache, coma, disorientation, seizures
  - Cardiac: flushed skin, VF, ↓BP
  - GI: absent
  - Respiratory: hypoventilation with hypoxia

METABOLIC AND RESPIRATORY ALKALOSIS
PATHOPHYSIOLOGY

- Metabolic alkalosis
  - Decreased strong acid or increased base, with compensatory CO_2 retention by lungs.
- Respiratory alkalosis
  - Hyperventilation and increased excretion of CO_2, with compensatory HCO_3 excretion by kidneys

LABORATORY

- Metabolic alkalosis

  - Increased serum pH
  - PCO_2 normal if uncompensated and increased if compensated
  - Increased HCO_3
  - Urine pH >6 if compensated

- Respiratory alkalosis

  - Increased serum pH
  - Decreased PCO_2
  - HCO_3 normal if uncompensated and decreased if compensated
  - Urine pH >6 if compensated

CAUSES

- Metabolic alkalosis

  - Excessive vomiting, gastric suctioning, diuretics, potassium deficit, excessive mineralocorticoids and $NaHCO_3$ intake

- Respiratory alkalosis

  - Hyperventilation associated with hypoxia, pulmonary embolus, exercise, anxiety, pain, and fever
  - Encephalopathy, septicemia, brain injury, salicylate overdose, mechanical hyperventilation

SYMPTOMS

- Metabolic alkalosis

  - Neuromuscular: dizziness, confusion, nervousness, anxiety, tremors, muscle cramping, tetany, tingling, seizures
  - Cardiac: tachycardia and arrhythmias
  - GI: nausea, vomiting, anorexia
  - Respiratory: compensatory hypoventilation

- Respiratory alkalosis

  - Neuro/muscular: light-headedness, confusion, lethargy
  - Cardiac: tachycardia and arrhythmias.
  - GI: epigastric pain, nausea, and vomiting
  - Respiratory: hyperventilation

Thermoregulation

NEUTRAL THERMAL ENVIRONMENT

A **neutral thermal environment** (NTE) is a place in which the infant's body temperature is maintained within a normal range without alterations in metabolic rate or increased oxygen consumption (i.e., environmental temperature in which oxygen consumption and glucose consumption are lowest). Infants who are in an NTE are not utilizing energy to maintain their body temperature in the normal range. Just because an infant has a normal body temperature does not mean he/she is in an NTE. The infant may still be utilizing mechanisms, such as non-shivering thermogenesis, to maintain body temperatures, as evidenced by increased oxygen consumption and poor weight gain over time. Charts are commercially available that outline the appropriate NTE for infants based on current weight and birth weight.

NON-SHIVERING THERMOGENESIS

Non-shivering thermogenesis (NST) is the major route of rapid increase of body temperature in response to cold stress in the term neonate. NST is the oxidation of brown fat to create heat. Brown adipose tissue contains a high concentration of stored triglycerides, a rich capillary network, and is controlled by the sympathetic nervous system. Brown fat cells have a rich supply of mitochondria that are unique, in that when fat is metabolized ATP is not produced, but instead heat is created. Temperature regulation is controlled by the posterior hypothalamus. When a cold body temperature is detected, the posterior hypothalamus responds by triggering the adrenal glands to release norepinephrine and the pituitary gland to release thyroxine. Both norepinephrine and thyroxine stimulate NST. Brown adipose production begins around 26 to 28 weeks of gestation and continues until 3 to 5 weeks after delivery. Premature infants have limited amounts of brown fat and limited ability to create heat via NST.

HEAT TRANSFER MECHANISMS

There are four **heat transfer mechanisms** to consider when caring for a neonate, especially a premature one: conduction, convection, radiation, and evaporation. Mechanisms include:

- **Conduction**: The transfer of heat between solid objects of different temperatures in contact with each other. Heat is transferred from the body of the infant to a cold surface they may come into contact with, such as a scale. Care should be taken to make sure the scales are warmed before use. Conduction can also be used to warm the infant by placing a warmed blanket next to the skin to conduct the warmth to the infant.
- **Convection**: The transfer of heat through air currents to the air moving around and across an infant's body. Incubators use convection of warm air being pumped into the incubator to keep an infant warm. Heat can be lost this way if a cool draft is allowed to be near the infant. (Continued)

Radiation and evaporation are two additional heat transfer mechanisms:

- **Radiation**: Heat transferred between two objects not in contact with each other. This is the transfer of heat through emission of infrared rays. Radiant warming beds use this mechanism to warm the infant. Heat loss occurs when an infant is in an incubator and the walls of the incubator are cooler than body temperature. The neonate in an incubator with this situation will lose body heat through radiation from his body to the cooler walls despite the warm air being pumped in.

- **Evaporation**: Loss of heat occurring when moisture evaporates from the surface of the skin. Evaporation is the result of conversion of liquid into a vapor and is a major concern at birth, as a wet infant can experience a 3-degree drop in body temperature in only about 10 minutes. Thus, drying and replacing wet linens with warm and dry ones is critical at birth.

EVAPORATIVE HEAT LOSS AND HUMIDITY RELATED TO PRETERM INFANTS

Evaporative heat loss occurs when moisture vaporizes from the skin of an infant. In infants born younger than 31 weeks gestation, evaporative heat loss is greatly enhanced by the poor keratinization of the infant's skin. Poor keratinization makes skin highly permeable, which promotes both fluid and heat loss. This permeability decreases 7-10 days after birth. The amount of evaporation is dependent on the relative humidity of the environment. The more **humid the environment**, the more that evaporation and its associated heat loss are suppressed. A dry environment promotes evaporative heat and fluid loss through the skin. An incubator with humidity controls should be used for infants who are vulnerable to evaporative heat loss. Infants prone to temperature instability should be kept in a highly humid environment.

HEAT LOSS IN PRETERM INFANTS

Preterm infants have not yet developed many of the features that full term infants use to help protect them from heat loss. The characteristics that make premature infants especially vulnerable to cold stress include:

- Larger surface area to body mass ratio that allows for quicker transfer of body heat to the environment.
- Decreased amounts of subcutaneous fat that provides insulation from heat loss.
- Decreased amounts of brown fat used for non-shivering thermogenesis.
- Immature skin that is not completely keratinized is more permeable to evaporative water and heat loss.
- Inability to flex the body to conserve heat.
- Limited control of skin blood flow mechanisms that conserve heat.

MINIMIZING HEAT LOSS

At delivery, **minimize heat loss** while evaluating the newborn by following these steps:

- Dry the infant thoroughly (including hair) to minimize evaporative heat loss, and remove wet towels.
- Place a cap on the infant's head, as the head is the most significant area of heat loss.
- When the infant is to be weighed, cover the scales with a warm cloth to minimize conductive heat loss.
- Place the infant in a warm environment such as:
  - Skin-to-skin contact with mother, and cover them with a warm blanket.
  - Bundled in warm blankets and given to the mother to hold.
  - Underneath a preheated warmer for further evaluation or resuscitation.

Minimizing heat loss is especially important if the newborn is premature or has intrauterine growth restriction, but full-term newborns also suffer if they become chilled.

SKIN TEMPERATURE PROBES

Skin temperature probes are often used to monitor the temperature of the infant in an Isolette or radiant warmer. Incorrect placement of the probe can alter the reading, causing the warming device to deliver too much or too little heat. The temperature probe should not be placed over a bony area of the body or over an area where brown adipose tissue is abundant. Brown adipose tissue is abundant around the neck, the midscapular region of the back, the mediastinum and organs in the thoracic cavity, kidneys, and adrenal glands. A common probe placement area for an infant who is supine is over the liver. If the probe is not making good skin contact, it will indicate that the infant is cold, and the warmer will deliver increased amounts of heat, possibly causing hyperthermia. If the probe is underneath the infant, it may indicate an artificially warm temperature and decrease heat to the infant, causing hypothermia.

COLD STRESS/HYPOTHERMIA

Cold stress/hypothermia in the neonate is a body temperature measurement of less than 36.5 °C rectally with associated symptoms. Preterm neonates are especially vulnerable to cold stress, as they have limited ability to intrinsically create or conserve body heat. They do not shiver, have limited ability to constrict superficial blood vessels and have limited amounts of both subcutaneous and brown fat. Signs of cold stress include:

- Body is cool to touch.
- Central cyanosis and acrocyanosis.
- Mottling of skin.
- Poor feeding, weak suck, increased gastric residuals, and abdominal distension.
- Bradycardia.
- Shallow respirations with tachypnea.
- Restlessness and irritability.
- Apnea.
- Lethargy and decreased activity.
- Weak cry.
- Hypoglycemia.
- Central nervous system depression with hypotonia.
- Edema.

THERMOREGULATION TO TREAT HYPOTHERMIA

There are a number of steps in the **treatment of hypothermia**:

1. Determine if the cause of hypothermia is from an abnormal physiological process in the infant or from environmental conditions.
2. Rewarm the infant slowly, because too rapid rewarming may result in apnea or hypotension.
3. Maintain the ambient temperature at 1 to 1.5 °C higher than the infant's temperature. Oxygen consumption is not elevated when the difference between the skin temperature and the environmental air temperature is less than 1.5 °C.
4. Increase the air temperature by approximately 1 °C every hour until the infant's temperature is in the normal range and stable.
5. Warm IV fluids with a blood-warming device prior to infusion, to enhance warming of the child.
6. Closely monitor the infant's blood glucose levels, vital signs, and urinary output during rewarming.

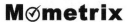

HYPERTHERMIA

Hyperthermia (rectal temperature greater than 37.0 °C) can be caused by excessive heat from an external source (such as a radiant warmer set too high) or internally from a hypermetabolic state (such as a fever):

External heat source	Hypermetabolic
Core temperature < skin temperature.	Core temperature > skin temperature.
Skin warm and flushed.	Skin cool to touch.

Infants who are physiologically competent attempt to cool themselves when hyperthermia is caused by an external heat source by an extended posture, diaphoresis, and flushed, warm skin. Hyperthermia in the neonate can cause increased metabolic demands, vasodilatation, and increased fluid loss. An increased metabolic demand leads to an increased oxygen requirement, hypoxia, cyanosis, and breathing irregularities, such as tachypnea. Increased glucose consumption leads to hypoglycemia and its associated signs (jitteriness, lethargy, vomiting, or seizures). Peripheral vasodilatation helps cool the infant but may cause tachycardia and hypotension. Increased fluid losses contribute to tachycardia and hypotension. Signs of shock may develop with lethargy and decreased urine output. Dehydration may also cause electrolyte abnormalities.

INCUBATORS

The goal of placing an infant in an **incubator** is to provide a neutral thermal environment (NTE) that places minimal stress on the infant. Most incubators are rigid, box-like structures like an Isolette, in which an infant is kept in a controlled environment to receive medical care. The infant is allowed to grow and mature here before being transitioned to the more "uncontrolled" environment of an open crib. Features that incubators possess that enhance the production of an NTE include a heater, a fan to circulate warmed air, and a humidity control. They also usually have a way to increase the oxygen content of the environment and ports to allow for nursing care without removing the infant. A servo-control is used in conjunction with a temperature-sensing thermistor that is attached to the infant to help regulate the infant's temperature within a set range. Some incubators may have double walls that lessen radiant heat loss. Infants who are in need of close monitoring are not placed in an incubator, but instead are placed under a radiant warmer with minimal covering. This allows the nurse to monitor the infant's skin color and breathing patterns more closely.

RADIANT WARMERS

Radiant warmers are devices that provide overhead heat directly to the infant. Radiant heaters provide an area for direct observation and free access to the infant, which is very useful in the initial evaluation and resuscitation (if necessary) of the newborn, or for procedures such as intubation or line placement. Radiant heat devices work best if the room temperature is kept above 25 °C. Two problems related to radiant warmers include:

- Promote dehydration if an infant is placed under them for a prolonged amount of time, especially if the infant is premature.
- Risk overheating the infant or cause first-degree burns.

Temperature sensors must be appropriately placed and the infant's temperature monitored frequently to ensure the infant is not being over or under heated.

SERVOCONTROL

The **servocontrol** is a thermistor probe used to monitor the temperature of the infant in an incubator or radiant warmer. The servocontrol is essentially the automatic thermostat that adjusts the environmental temperature in response to the infant's body temperature. Typically, the infant's temperature should be maintained at 36 to 36.5° C. Incorrect placement of the probe can alter the reading, causing the warming device to deliver too much or too little heat. The servocontrol should avoid a bony area of the body or an area where brown adipose tissue is abundant (neck, midscapular region, mediastinum, and organs in the thoracic cavity, kidneys, and adrenal glands). If the infant is supine, the probe is placed on the abdomen at the midpoint between the xiphoid process and the umbilicus. If prone, the probe is placed over either flank. If in a radiant warmer, a special foil shield should protect the probe. If the probe is not making good skin contact, it will indicate that the infant is cold, and the warmer will deliver increased amounts of heat, possibly causing hyperthermia. If the probe is underneath the infant, it may indicate an artificially warm temperature and decrease heat to the infant, causing hypothermia.

Neurodevelopmental Care

NEUROBEHAVIORAL DEVELOPMENT

Terms related to **neurobehavioral development**:

- **Habituation**: A decreasing response to repeated stimuli. For example, if a child is exposed to repeated sounds, the child will over time become used to the sound and show less reaction.
- **Motor organization**: Motor organization involves 3 different levels: (1) the spinal cord (which mediates automatic movement and reflexes), (2) brain stem (which includes the medial descending systems that control body movement and antigravity reflexes and the lateral descending systems that control voluntary limb movements) (3) the cerebral cortex (which regulates movement).
- **State organization**: The brain has the ability to respond differently in different states or conditions, suggesting that the neonate's brain is active and not just passive.
- **Sensory/Interaction capabilities**: The ability to respond to stimuli and to interact with the environment and others. The interactions the neonate has after birth with others (dyadic interactions) help the child to learn patterns of interactions and responses.

SLEEP STATES

Infants spend a high percentage of their time in **sleep states**. Sleep periods are divided into active sleep or quiet sleep by observing the infant's behavior:

- **Quiet sleep** is restorative and fosters anabolic growth. Quiet sleep is associated with increased cell mitosis and replication, lowered oxygen consumption, and the release of growth hormone. During quiet sleep, the infant appears relaxed, moves minimally, and breathes smoothly and regularly. The eyelids are still. The infant only responds to intense stimuli during quiet sleep.
- **Active sleep** is associated with processing and storing of information. Rapid eye movement (REM sleep) occurs during active sleep, but it is unknown if newborn infants are able to dream. During active sleep, the infant moves occasionally and breathes irregularly. Eye movements can be seen beneath the eyelids. Infants spend most of their sleep time in active sleep, and it usually precedes wakening.

AWAKE STATES

Infants have different levels of consciousness in the 4 **awake states**. Infants respond differently to outside stimuli and interaction from caregivers, depending on which state they are in:

- **Drowsy:** This is characterized by variable activity, mild startles, and smooth movement. There is some facial movement. Eyes open and close, breathing is irregular, and response to stimuli may be delayed.
- **Quiet alert:** The infant rarely moves, breathing is regular, and the infant focuses intently on individuals or objects that are within focal range, widening eyes. Face appears bright and alert, breathing is regular, and the infant focuses on stimuli.
- **Active alert:** The infant moves frequently and has much facial movement although face not as bright and alert, eyes may have a dull glaze, breathing is irregular, and there are variable responses to outside stimuli.
- **Crying:** Characterized by grimacing, eyes shut, irregular breathing, increased movement with color changes and marked response to both internal and external stimuli.

STAGES OF SITTING IN INFANT DEVELOPMENT

The newborn will begin to show signs of preparedness to begin the **sitting process** at 4 months of age, in conjunction with the ability to stabilize the head. At this point the infant will be able to sit with help from parents or a seat. This action will then progress to unassisted sitting any time between 6-9 months, but the infant will still require assistance from the caretaker (pull to sit) to get into the sitting position. The more practice the infant has in the sitting position, the quicker he/she will adapt to the position and gain the muscles and stability to sit without the assistance of a parent or seat/stabilizing cushion. In combination with tummy time, sitting helps build muscles that lead to the next stage of development: crawling.

BRAZELTON NEONATAL BEHAVIORAL ASSESSMENT SCALE

The **Brazelton Neonatal Behavioral Assessment Scale** is a multi-dimensional scale that is used to assess a neonate's state, temperament, and behavioral patterns. It includes the assessment of 18 reflexes, 28 behaviors, and 6 other characteristics. It is usually completed on day 3 with an attempt to elicit the most positive response, usually when the infant is comforted and in a quiet dim room. Scoring correlates to the child's awake or sleep state. Infants are scored according to response in many areas, including:

- **Habituation**: Ability to diminish response to repeat stimuli.
- **Visual and auditory orientation:** Ability to respond to stimuli, fixate, and follow a visual object.
- **Motor activity:** Assessment of body tone in various activities.
- Variations: Changes in color, state, activity, alertness, and excitement during the exam.
- **Self-quieting activities:** Frequency and speed of self-calming activities, such as sucking on their hand, putting their hand to their mouth, and focusing on an object or sound.
- **Social behaviors:** Ability to cuddle, engage, and enjoy physical contact.

KANGAROO CARE

Dr. Edgar Ray invented **kangaroo care** in the late 1970's in Bogotá, Columbia, when morbidity and mortality rates rose in his NICU, but he had limited technological resources. Kangaroo care consists of placing the infant, after drying and warming, in minimal clothing in an upright position on the mother's bare chest between her breasts. This allows for skin-to-skin contact with the infant's head next to the mother's heart. A precipitous drop was noted in premature infant mortality after this method of care was instigated. The concept is to provide the neonate with closeness similar to that experienced with the mother while in the womb. Kangaroo care is maintained for as long as the neonate allows. Preterm infants attached to ventilators and IV infusions also benefit from kangaroo care. There are physiological and psychological benefits for both the neonate and the mother. Enhanced bonding between the neonate and the mother, shorter hospital stays, low cost, and decreased morbidity and mortality are all documented benefits.

Some specific benefits of kangaroo care for the mother, the neonate, and the institution are listed below:

- **Mother's Benefits**
  - o Enhanced bonding with the infant.
  - o Increased production of milk with higher rates of successful breastfeeding.
  - o Increased confidence in caring for the infant.
  - o Increased opportunity for teaching and assessing maternal care by nursing staff.
- **Neonate's Benefits**
  - o Regulation of temperature, heart and respiratory rates.
  - o Calming effect with decreased stress.
  - o Decreased episodes of apnea.
  - o Increased weight gain.
  - o Enhanced bonding with the mother.
  - o Fewer nosocomial infections.
- **Institutional Benefits**
  - o Earlier discharge from hospital.
  - o Decreased morbidity and mortality (especially in developing countries).
  - o Decreased use of financial resources.

PROVIDING WARMTH

Infants have poor temperature regulation ability, particularly preterm infants who lack brown fat, which is one of the body's tools to regulate body temperature, so **providing warmth** is critical as a component of resuscitation. An infant who is just seconds old and wet will need aggressive measures to keep it warm while any resuscitation efforts are being initiated. Infants lose heat through their head so one of the first steps should be to place a hat on the head. The infant should be placed under a radiant heater and vigorous drying with warmed blankets should begin. Often this stimulation, drying and warming is all that is needed to establish a regular respiration pattern in the neonate. Preterm infants weighing <1500 grams should be placed in a plastic bag (made specifically for this purpose) up to the height of the shoulders to prevent cold shock. A term infant with no apparent distress can be placed on the mother's chest and covered with a warm blanket.

STRESS RELATED TO LIGHT

Light is a necessary component of caring for both the sick and healthy neonate in the delivery room and nursery. Adequate lighting is required to evaluate the at-risk neonate, to assess color, to complete procedures such as intubation, or to give medications. Light discourages the growth of pathogens. However, constant bright light interferes with the development of natural diurnal rhythms because it arouses the central nervous system and stresses the infant. Controlling light helps to stabilize the infant. Some simple methods to protect the neonate from light over-stimulation and to establish a normal sleep cycle include:

- Reducing overhead light levels when direct visualization is not necessary.
- Covering incubator hoods to reduce light entering the incubator.
- Dimming the lights at night to help establish a natural day/night pattern (circadian rhythm).

STRESS RELATED TO NOISE

Excessive **noise** causes agitation in both term and especially preterm neonates. The preterm neonate has less ability to self-calm, and over-stimulation results in decompensation, as demonstrated by increased oxygen requirements and increased apnea and bradycardia episodes. The American Academy of Pediatrics (AAP) recommends noise levels in the nursery and NICU be kept at **≤45 decibels**. A normal speaking voice is between 50 to 60 decibels. Noise levels above 80 to 85 decibels damage the cochlea and cause hearing loss in adults. To keep noise acceptably low:

- Turn radios/TVs off or down.
- Designate a daily quiet time.
- Close incubator portholes gently, because closing a plastic porthole can spike the decibel level more than 80 dB.
- *Whisper* — avoid speaking loudly.
- Remove bubbling water from ventilator tubing.
- Educate parents about the deleterious effects of over-stimulating their infant with loud noises.

ENVIRONMENTAL STRESSORS AND "TIME OUT"

Premature neonates have a very limited ability to deal with **environmental stressors,** but these stressors can affect all neonates. Signs of stress in neonates include:

- Color changes, such as mottling or cyanosis.
- Episodes of apnea and bradycardia.
- Activity changes, such as tremors, twitches, frantic activity, arching, and gaze averting.
- Flaccid posture (sagging trunk, extremities and face).
- Easy fatigability.

When the infant shows signs of stress, a **"time out"** recovery period is indicated:

- Stop the activity causing the stress.
- Reduce unnecessary stimuli, e.g., lower the lights and postpone non-essential manipulation of the neonate.
- Give the neonate a chance to calm or soothe himself.
- Bundle the neonate and place him/her in a comforting, side-lying position with the shoulders drawn forward and the hands brought to midline.

NON-NUTRITIVE SUCKING

Nonnutritive sucking occurs when an infant sucks on an item such as a pacifier, or his/her own fist. Nonnutritive sucking is not associated with nutritional intake, but it is an important method of self-quieting and begins in the uterus at about 29 weeks of gestation. Extremely premature infants often lack basic neurodevelopmental capabilities, and cannot coordinate sucking, swallowing, and breathing simultaneously. Typically, the ability to suck and swallow in a coordinated fashion is not present until 32 to 34 weeks of gestation. Premature infants should be encouraged to perform non-nutritive sucking during the gavage feeding process if they can accomplish it. Benefits of nonnutritive sucking include:

- Improved digestion of enteral feeds because digestive enzyme release is stimulated.
- Facilitated development of coordinated nutritive sucking behavior.
- Calming of the distressed infant.

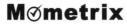

POSITIONING OF THE PREMATURE NEONATE

Correct positioning of the premature neonate minimizes outside stimuli and mimics the enclosed and calming environment of the womb, helping with the transition to extrauterine life:

- Place the neonate in a flexed position, with his hands close to midline and near his face.
- Create a nest of blankets or pillows to:
  o Help block out light and noise.
  o Give him the impression of a closed environment.
  o Minimize abnormal molding of the head from prolonged pressure on one side.
- Cover the incubator to further keep out sound and light.
- Place the neonate in the prone position (on his stomach) to help to stabilize the chest wall, improves ventilation, and increases the amount of time an infant is in quiet sleep. However, infants should be placed supine (on the back) most of the time, to decrease the chance of SIDS.

Substance Exposure in Utero

FETAL ALCOHOL SYNDROME

Fetal alcohol syndrome (FAS) is a syndrome of birth defects that develop as the result of maternal ingestion of alcohol. Fetal alcohol spectrum disorders (FASD) is an umbrella diagnosis that includes FAS along with infants impacted by alcohol in utero that do not meet the full FAS criteria. Despite campaigns to inform the public, women continue to drink during pregnancy, but no safe amount of alcohol ingestion has been determined. FAS includes:

- **Facial abnormalities**: Hypoplastic (underdeveloped) maxilla, micrognathia (undersized jaw), hypoplastic philtrum (groove beneath the nose), short palpebral fissures (eye slits between upper and lower lids).
- **Neurological deficits**: May include microcephaly, intellectual disability, and motor delay, hearing deficits. Learning disorders may include problems with visual-spatial and verbal learning, attention disorders, delayed reaction times.
- **Growth restriction**: Prenatal growth deficit persists with slow growth after birth.
- **Behavioral problems**: Irritability and hyperactivity. Poor judgment in behavior may relate to deficit in executive functions.

Indication of brain damage without the associated physical abnormalities is referred to as alcohol-related neurodevelopmental disorder (ARND).

FETAL EXPOSURE TO TOBACCO/NICOTINE

Tobacco smoke contains many substance known to be detrimental to a person's health. When a pregnant woman smokes, her fetus is exposed to carbon monoxide, nicotine, and hydrogen cyanide that all cross the placenta. Carbon monoxide displaces oxygen from hemoglobin, resulting in decreased oxygen delivery to the fetus. Exposure increases risk of miscarriage and perinatal death. Infants exposed *in utero* to tobacco may have the following problems:

- Decreased length, weight, and head circumference.
- Increased rates of congenital birth defects, such as cleft palate or lip, limb reduction defects, and urinary tract anomalies.
- Increased incidence of placenta previa, placental abruption, and preterm birth.

If smoking continues after delivery, these further detrimental effects may occur:

- Sudden infant death syndrome.
- Increased infant respiratory tract infections and childhood asthma.
- Behavioral problems in later childhood.

FETAL EXPOSURE TO MARIJUANA, PHENCYCLIDINE (PCP), AND MDMA

Marijuana, phencyclidine (PCP), and methylenedioxymethamphetamine (MDMA or ecstasy) are popular and "club" drugs that may be used by some women during pregnancy:

- **Marijuana**: This is often used along with alcohol and tobacco, so effects are difficult to assess, but there do not appear to be teratogenic effects; however, some studies report exposure can result in fine tremors, irritability, and prolonged startle response for the first 12 months after birth.
- **PCP**: One of the biggest problems with PCP is that mothers may have an overdose or psychotic response that can result in hypertension, hyperthermia, and coma, compromising the fetus.
- **MDMA**: Ecstasy is a popular club drug that is frequently used by teenagers and young adults. There is no clear evidence regarding effects on the fetus although some research suggests it may cause long-term impairments in learning.

FETAL EXPOSURE TO AMPHETAMINES

Amphetamines are a class of drugs that cause CNS stimulation. The most commonly abused amphetamine is methamphetamine. Maternal use of these substances causes hypertension and tachycardia, which can cause miscarriage, abruptio placentae, and premature delivery. Vasoconstriction affects placental vessels, decreasing circulation, nutrition, and oxygen to the fetus. Methamphetamines can cross the placental barrier and cause fetal hypertension and prenatal strokes and damage to the heart and other organs. The neonate is commonly small for gestational age, often ≤5 pounds, full term but ≤10 percentile for weight, with shortened length and smaller head circumference. The neonate in withdrawal from maternal amphetamine use will suffer abnormal sleep patterns, often characterized by lethargy and excessive sleeping during the first few weeks, poor feeding, tremors, diaphoresis, miosis, frantic fist sucking, high-pitched crying, fever, excessive yawning, and hyperreflexia.

FETAL EXPOSURE TO HEROIN

Heroin is a highly addictive, opioid narcotic that is a common drug of abuse. Heroin users are at increased risk of poor nutrition, iron deficiency anemia and preeclampsia-eclampsia, all negatively affecting the fetus. Infants with prenatal heroin exposure display symmetric intrauterine growth restriction (IUGR) and are often born prematurely. About 60-80% of these infants will undergo neonatal abstinence syndrome (NAS). Heroin has a relatively short half-life and symptoms of NAR typically begin 48-72 hours after delivery. Several different body systems are affected by NAS and include:

CNS Dysfunction	GI Dysfunction	Miscellaneous Signs
High-pitched cry hyperactive.	Poor feeding.	Frequent yawning.
Reflexes increased muscle.	Periods of frantic sucking or rooting.	Sneezing multiple times.
Irritability.	Vomiting.	Sweating.
Tremors.	Loose or watery stools.	Fever.
	Vomiting.	Tachypnea.

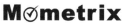

FETAL EXPOSURE TO METHADONE

Methadone is commonly used to treat women who are addicted to opioids, such as heroin or prescriptive narcotics, as it blocks withdrawal symptoms and drug craving. An associated risk is that methadone crosses the placental barrier and exposes the fetus to the drug. Many female heroin users are of reproductive age and methadone is often administered to pregnant women to decrease dangers associated with heroin, such as fluctuating levels of drug and exposure to hepatitis and HIV from sharing of needles. Exposure to methadone may result in miscarriage, stillbirth, intrauterine growth restriction, fetal distress, and low birth rate although symptoms are usually less severe than with heroin. However, if the mother takes methadone and other drugs, this can compound the adverse effects. Additionally, sudden withdrawal from methadone may cause preterm labor or death of the fetus, so methadone should be monitored carefully.

FETAL EXPOSURE TO COCAINE

Cocaine/crack (freebase cocaine) is a nonopioid substance that readily crosses the placenta through simple diffusion. One of the most potent properties of cocaine is the ability of it to act as a vasoconstrictor. When a mother uses cocaine, the blood supply to the placenta is severely compromised when the vessels constrict, compromising blood flow and resulting in growth restriction and hypoxia. Cocaine also causes a programmed cell death (known as apoptosis) in the heart muscle cells of the fetus, resulting in cardiac dysfunction for the fetus. Maternal cocaine use increases the risk of premature birth and causes serious consequences for the neonate after birth. Maternal cocaine use can cause cerebral infarctions, nonduodenal intestinal atresia, anal atresia, NEC, defects of the limbs, and genitourinary defects. Cocaine stimulates the central nervous system by limiting the uptake of certain neurotransmitters norepinephrine, serotonin, and dopamine. Cocaine has a direct toxic effect on the nervous system, so the infant will exhibit extreme irritability and tremors followed by sluggish, lethargic behavior.

FETAL EXPOSURE TO COMMON PRESCRIPTION/OTC DRUGS

Many **OTC and prescription drugs** have teratogenic effects on the developing fetus and can result in congenital abnormalities, growth restriction, intellectual disability, carcinogenesis, mutagenesis, and miscarriage. The degree of damage relates to multiple factors, such as the amount of drug reaching the fetus, the developmental period during which the drug is taken, and the duration. There are some recognizable syndromes:

- **Fetal warfarin (Coumadin®) syndrome** (exposure 7-12 weeks): Nasal hypoplasia, laryngomalacia, atrial septal defects, patent ductus arteriosis, eye, ear, and skull abnormalities, intellectual disabilities and growth restriction, brachydactyly, and scoliosis. Exposure during 2nd and 3rd trimester may result in eye abnormalities (cataracts, optic atrophy), microphthalmia (eyes stop developing resulting in abnormally small eyes), fetal/maternal hemorrhage, and microcephaly,
- **Fetal hydantoin (Dilantin®) syndrome** (exposure 1st trimester): Facial dysmorphism, microcephaly, underdeveloped nails (hands and feet), cleft left/palate, and developmental delays ranging from mild to severe.
- **Fetal valproate (Depakote®) syndrome** (exposure 1st trimester): Facial dysmorphism, spina bifida, CNS and cardiac abnormalities, and delay in development.

Some drugs are classified as high risk (FDA classification D), but use is acceptable if the mother has a life-threatening illness or other drugs are not available, so neonates may exhibit adverse effects.

Drugs with high risk include and their adverse effects on the fetus/infant include:

- **ACE inhibitors** (2nd and 3rd trimesters): Skull and pulmonary hypoplasia, renal tubular dysplasia, and oligohydramnios.
- **Carbamazepine** (1st trimester): Craniofacial defects, neural tube defects, restriction of growth, and hypoplasia of fingernails.
- **Antineoplastic alkylating drugs** (1st to 3rd trimesters): Eye disorders, including microphthalmia and cataracts, cardiac defects, renal agenesis, and cardiac abnormalities.
- **Iodides** (3rd trimester): Thyroid disorders, including goiter, and fetal hypothyroidism.
- **Methimazole** (1st trimester): Aplasia cutis.
- **Lithium** (1st trimester): Ebstein anomaly, various cardiac abnormalities.
- **Tetracycline** (2nd and 3rd trimesters): Yellow discoloration of teeth. Weakening of fetal bones and dysplasia of tooth enamel.

Some drugs are classified as extremely high risk (FDA classification X), and these drugs should not be used with women who are pregnant or might become pregnant because fetal risk outweighs benefits to mother:

- **Androgens** (1st trimester): Female fetus will become masculinized.
- **Retinoids** – isotretinoin, acitretin, tretinoin, etretinate (1st trimester): Multiple deformities of heart, ears, face, limbs, & liver, cognitive impairment, thymic hypoplasia, microcephalus, hydrocephalus, microtia, and miscarriage.
- **Thalidomide** (days 34-60): Multiple facial, intestinal, cardiac, limb abnormalities, including lack of limbs and limb reductions, and deafness.
- **Vitamin A** (>18,000 IU/day): Multiple craniofacial deformities, microtia, CAN and cardiac abnormalities, atresia of bowel, limb reductions, and defects of urinary tract.

SUBUTEX

Subutex (buprenorphine) is indicated for pregnant women who are opioid or heroin dependent. This medication is often prescribed to patients at risk for experiencing the withdrawal symptoms from their addiction, which can be severe and inhibit the mother's ability to fully detox. Subutex is an opioid agonist that helps the patient avoid withdrawal symptoms by occupying opioid receptors (therefore quenching the addiction) without producing a high. While the use of Subutex has not been guaranteed as safe during pregnancy, it has been proven to be safer than opioid use during pregnancy and can help the user in the detoxification process. While there is still a risk of the newborn experiencing NAS (Neonatal Abstinence Syndrome) after birth with the maternal use of Subutex, this has been deemed less harmful than the impact of opioid use on the fetus.

NAS AND WITHDRAWAL ASSOCIATED WITH MATERNAL SUBSTANCE ABUSE

Neonatal abstinence syndrome (NAS) includes the manifestations of withdrawal that a neonate undergoes after exposure to drugs while *in utero.* These may vary somewhat depending on the type and extent of substance abuse, which may include prescription narcotics, heroin, antidepressants, and benzodiazepines. NAS is more readily treated if the mother's substance abuse was controlled with drugs such as methadone and buprenorphine. Buprenorphine causes less severe NAS than methadone. Substance abuse may result in *in utero* growth restriction, abruptio placentae, fetal cardiac arrhythmias, preterm labor and delivery, and fetal death. Neonates often have low birth weight, small head circumference, tremors, seizures, diarrhea, and hypertonic reflexes. They may feed poorly, so they may need high-caloric formula, and may cry excessively and sleep poorly. The infant may receive drugs (morphine, methadone, and buprenorphine) to relieve withdrawal symptoms. Dehydrated infants (from diarrhea) may require IV fluids. Swaddling, kangaroo care, and maintaining a quiet dimly lit environment may help to soothe the infant.

MANAGING SYMPTOMS OF INTRAUTERINE DRUG EXPOSURE
HIGH-PITCHED CRYING AND INABILITY TO SLEEP

Interventions for high-pitched crying include the following:

- Keep room quiet with low light.
- Swaddle the infant securely in a flexed position with the arms close to the body.
- Hold infant close to body.
- Rock swaddled infant slowly and rhythmically.
- Walk with swaddled infant held close.
- Offer pacifier, possibly with sugar solution, if acceptable.
- Give a warm bath.
- Play soft music.
- Placing the infant in a dark room with no stimulation at all for a period of time may be effective if other methods fail.

Interventions for inability to sleep include the following:

- Decrease environmental stimuli and maintain quiet.
- Waterbed or sheepskin.
- Feed frequently in small amounts.

NASAL STUFFINESS, POOR FEEDING, AND REGURGITATION

Interventions for nasal stuffiness/sneezing include the following:

- Aspirate nasopharynx as needed.
- Feed slowly and give time for rest between sucking.
- Monitor respirations.

Interventions for poor feeding and frantic sucking of fingers/fist include the following:

- Feed small frequent amounts with enteral feedings if necessary.
- Weigh daily.
- Provide nonnutritive sucking with pacifier to relieve frantic sucking.

Interventions for regurgitation include the following:

- Weigh frequently and monitor fluids and electrolytes.
- Observe for dehydration and provide IV fluids as needed.
- Place supine with head elevated after feedings.

HYPERTONICITY, DIARRHEA, AND TREMOR/SEIZURES

Interventions for hypertonicity include the following:

- Monitor temperature and decrease environmental temperature if infant's temperature >37.6 °C.
- Change infant's position frequently to avoid pressure sores.
- Place on sheepskin or waterbed to prevent pressure.

Interventions for diarrhea include the following:

- Change diaper frequently and cleanse skin with mild soap and water. Apply skin barrier as needed.
- Expose irritated skin to air.

Interventions for tremor/seizures include the following:

- Decrease environmental stimuli and handling.
- Change position frequently.
- Observe for scratches, blistering, or abrasions.
- Place on sheepskin or waterbed to reduce friction and pressure.
- Maintain patent airway and observe for apnea.
- Monitor for hyperthermia.

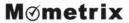

Infection and Immunity

NEONATE IMMUNITY

Infants (especially preterm) have **increased susceptibility to infection** when compared to older children and adults because of immaturity or deficiencies in their immune systems:

- **Cellular immunity**: Neutrophils and macrophages in the neonate are deficient in chemotaxis and not as effective in killing invading bacteria. Reserves of neutrophils are easily depleted in neonates.
- **Humoral immunity**: Some passage of immunoglobulin G (IgG) occurs from the mother to the fetus, but mostly during the third trimester. In general, immunoglobulin levels are low. The neonate does not produce IgA until 2-5 weeks after birth. Complement activity is also immature in newborns, leaving them especially susceptible to Gram-negative organisms.
- **Barrier function**: The skin and mucous membranes, which normally act as barriers, are less effective in newborns. Prolonged invasive instrumentation (central lines or endotracheal tubes), associated with infants who are premature or those with complex congenital deformities, are other routes for infection.

HUMORAL IMMUNITY

Humoral immunity in neonates is mainly mediated by maternal transfer of Immunoglobulin G (IgG) that greatly increases after 32 weeks of gestation. Infants born prior 32 weeks have a significantly lower immunoglobulin level than term infants. Endogenous production of immunoglobulins does not begin until 24 weeks after birth, allowing serum immunoglobulin levels to trough until production begins. This trough further lowers the premature infant's ability to fight infections. The lower the infant's gestational age, the higher the incidence of neonatal sepsis. The risk of neonatal sepsis is 10 times higher in infants who weigh less than 2,500 grams, when compared to full term infants. Boost the premature infant's immunoglobulin level with intravenous IgG (IVIG) to prevent the acquisition of nosocomial infections or as adjunctive therapy in neonates with early onset sepsis. (Studies have shown mixed results with only minimal benefits.)

ANTIBODIES

Antibodies (immunoglobins) are proteins that aid in the fight against bacteria, viruses and toxins. These antibodies are created in response to the presence of antigens and/or are passed along from mother to fetus/newborn through pregnancy and breastfeeding. Immunoglobin tests are often indicated in the newborn to identify deficiencies.

Key immunoglobins in the infant include:

- **IgA:** Found in mucus membranes (respiratory and GI tract), saliva, tears but is also passed along to the infant through the human milk; prevents the colonization of pathogens.
- **IgG:** Most abundant; found in bodily fluids; respond to and protect against viral and bacterial infections; the only immunoglobin that passes through the placenta during pregnancy providing passive immunity to the fetus.
- **IgM:** Found in blood and lymph fluid; the "first responder" to new infections and primary infection fighter until IgG arrives.

NEUTROPHILS

Neutrophils are phagocytic white blood cells (WBC). Their granules kill bacteria and fungi by releasing lysozymes, peroxidase, and pyrogenic proteins. Normally, 50%-70% of WBC's are neutrophils. Their lifespan is three days. Reduced neutrophils (neutropenia) indicate infection or bone marrow suppression. A segmented neutrophil nucleus (seg) is a mature cell. A banded nucleus (band) is immature. To calculate the absolute neutrophil count (ANC), the hematologist adds the percentage of segs to the percentage of bands, and multiplies the result by the total white blood cell count. ANC by itself is a poor indicator of sepsis. A low ANC is more specific for identifying sepsis than an elevated ANC. **Normal neutrophil counts** change as the infant ages:

- At birth the lower limit of normal is 1,750 cells/mm^3
- At 12 hours it rises to 7,200 cells/mm^3
- At 72 hours it falls to 1,720 cells/mm^3

The immature to total neutrophil ratio (I:T) is a better indicator of sepsis than ANC. An I:T ratio greater than 0.2 indicates sepsis. The formula for calculating the I:T ratio is:

I:T = % immature neutrophils / (% immature neutrophils + %mature neutrophils)

CEREBROSPINAL FLUID LABORATORY PROFILE AND C-REACTIVE PROTEIN

CSF labs are used to diagnose bacterial meningitis. CSF findings suggestive of bacterial meningitis include:

- Decreased glucose.
- Elevated protein.
- White blood cells values in CSR greater than 100 WBC/dL.

A polymerase chain reaction assay test for Group B strep antigen in CSF is available. Antibiotics given to the mother prior to delivery or to the neonate prior to performing a lumbar puncture inhibit bacterial growth in cerebrospinal fluid (CSF), making the diagnosis dependent on other CSF parameters. Values may be more difficult to interpret in the premature neonate, as their blood brain barrier is more permeable.

C-reactive protein (CRP) is a blood marker for inflammation and is used to diagnose neonatal infections such as sepsis. If the CRP comes back as high, it indicates the possibility of sepsis, requiring further tests and treatment. CRP is created in the liver in reaction to infection, and takes about 48 hours to reach peak levels. CRP levels > 10mg/L are considered high in the neonate and worthy of furhter investigation.

SOURCES OF NEONATAL INFECTION

For the **neonate** there are three main categories of sources of infection:

- **Transplacental (Intrauterine):** This source of infection is a direct infection from the mother to the fetus prior to birth. Infections such as AIDS, Cytomegalovirus, Rubella, Syphilis and Toxoplasmosis are the most common types in this category.
- **Perinatal acquisition** during labor and delivery: This source of infection is at the time of birth rather than *in utero* and is a direct result of contact with a pathogen present on the mother at birth. Infections in this category include *Chlamydia*, Enterovirus, *Group B Streptococci,* Hepatitis B and Herpes.
- **Hospital acquisition** in the neonatal period is the third category. This is an infection that the infant did not have at birth but acquired from hospital personnel, equipment, the mother or visitors.

NOSOCOMIAL INFECTIONS IN THE NEONATAL UNIT

A **nosocomial infection** is acquired while in the hospital and is often responsible for late onset sepsis in neonates. The immature or compromised immune systems of premature neonates, combined with the frequent use of invasive ventilators, catheters, ventricular shunts, chest tubes, and IVs make neonates susceptible to nosocomial infections:

- Peripheral IVs are very common in neonates, and often require restarting because of their small and fragile veins. Appropriate aseptic technique is essential to lessen infections associated with peripheral IVs.
- Percutaneously inserted central catheters, commonly used in the NICU as they are more permanent than peripheral IVs, are also associated with nosocomial infections and should not be left in place longer than 21 days.

Pathogens commonly involved in nosocomial infections include coagulase negative *Staphylococcus* (CONS), *Klebsiella*, *Serratia*, *Enterobacter*, *Pseudomonas*, and *Candida*. Viral infections, such as respiratory syncytial virus (RSV), are usually introduced by parents and visitors. Frequent use of antibiotics contributes to the development of opportunistic bacteria and drug-resistant infections, such as Vancomycin-resistant *Enterococci* and methicillin-resistant *Staphylococcus aureus*.

HOSPITAL-ACQUIRED PNEUMONIA

KLEBSIELLA PNEUMONIAE

Klebsiella pneumoniae is a common cause of hospital-acquired infections of the urinary tract, surgical sites, and lower respiratory tract. *K. Pneumoniae* is a gram-negative member of the Enterobacteriaceae family and is part of the normal body flora. It can infect children of all ages but is most common in infants who are premature and/or in neonatal intensive care. Infants with invasive devices, such as those with mechanical ventilation, are at increased risk. There have been a number of outbreaks in neonatal units, especially with multi-drugs resistant forms, with the hands of health staff and the gastrointestinal tract of the infants providing reservoirs of bacteria. When the infection attacks the lungs, the *symptoms* include inflammatory changes that result in necrosis and hemorrhage, clogging the lungs with thick puro-sanguineous exudate. The disease spreads rapidly, with high fever and dyspnea. Mortality rates are high. *Treatment* includes antibiotic therapy (such as 3rd generation cephalosporins or quinolones) based on cultures and sensitivities.

PSEUDOMONAS AERUGINOSA

Hospital-acquired pneumonias (HAP) are far more lethal than community-acquired pneumonias (CAP), with HAP death rates of 20-40% and up to 90% if the infant is on mechanical ventilation, with **Pseudomonas aeruginosa** one of the most lethal (40-60% mortality) because it can invade blood vessels, resulting in hemorrhage. Most infections are spread by contact with contaminated hands of healthcare staff or from invasive devices, such as endotracheal tubes, and mechanical ventilators. *Symptoms* include fever, cough, bradycardia, and elevated WBC counts.

Treatment includes:

- Antibiotic therapy: Usually combinations of 2 antibiotics are given, such as piperacillin or ceftazidime AND gentamicin or ciprofloxacin (based on cultures). Vancomycin is generally avoided because of the rise of vancomycin-resistant organisms.
- Preventive measures include maintaining ventilated patients in 30° upright positions, universal precautions, and changing ventilator circuits as per protocol.

INFECTION CONTROL/UNIVERSAL PRECAUTIONS

There are a number of important steps in **infection control**:

- **Use standard precautions** including protection from all blood and body fluids and the use of gloves, face barriers, and gowns as needed to avoid being splashed with fluids. Hand washing remains central to infection control and should generally be with plain (not antimicrobial) soap or instant antiseptic. Hands should be washed with soap and water for 10-15 seconds between infant contacts but with antiseptic soap before invasive procedures.
- **Avoid overcrowding** by providing space of about 4-6 feet between neonates.
- **Avoid contaminating specimens** by using aseptic technique during collection and delivering specimens immediately to the laboratory.
- **Restrict infected staff** from working with neonates.
- **Cohort infants** with the same infectious organism and isolating them from other infants.
- **Maintain sterile technique** with invasive (IVs, central lines, or ventilator tubing) limits the introduction of potential pathogens.

VISITATION POLICIES FOR NEONATES WITH IMPAIRED IMMUNE SYSTEMS

Neonates with impaired immune systems often remain in the NICU post-partum and **visitation policies** must be in place to minimize infection risks and allow appropriate rest for the infant. That said, visitation is also important for the bonding process between the parents/siblings and the newborn. While some NICU policies have strict visitation policies, many do not consider parents/siblings as "visitors," allowing for a more family-centered approach to visitation and neonatal development. Visitation policies generally define who can visit, how many visitors can come at one time, and when visiting hours are available. For siblings, the general expectations are that they have not been exposed to any communicable diseases, they have no symptoms of a current acute illness, they have been prepared for what they will see in the visit, and that they will be supervised through the entirety of the visit.

VARICELLA ZOSTER

Chicken pox, caused by the **varicella zoster virus,** during the first 20 weeks of pregnancy can result in as infant with congenital varicella syndrome, which can cause a number of abnormalities of the skin, extremities, eyes, and central nervous system. Children are often unusually small with distinctive cicatrix scarring on the skin, and chorioretinitis. Brain abnormalities may include microcephaly, hydrocephalus, cortical atrophy, enlargement of the ventricles, and damage to the sympathetic nervous system. The child may suffer intellectual disabilities and developmental delays as well as lack of psychomotor coordination. If the mother is infected at the end of pregnancy and develops a rash from 5 days before to 2 days after delivery, the child may develop neonatal varicella, which poses of high risk to the child with mortality rates of about 30%. Vaccination prior to pregnancy is the best preventive. Premature neonates exposed after birth with ≤28 weeks gestation or ≥28 weeks if mother has no immunity should receive varicella zoster immunoglobulin (VZIG).

FETAL EXPOSURE TO RUBELLA

Women should always be vaccinated for **rubella** before becoming pregnant as exposure to the virus has devastating effects on the newborn. The mother may not experience any symptoms of the disease or only mild symptoms like mild respiratory problems or rash. If the rubella exposure is during the first 4 to 5 months of pregnancy, the consequences for the infant are greater. Infants exposed to this virus *in utero* can develop a set of symptoms known as congenital rubella syndrome. This syndrome includes all or some of the following signs and symptoms:

- Intrauterine growth restriction (IUGR).
- Deafness.
- Cataracts.
- Jaundice.
- Purpura.
- Hepatosplenomegaly.
- Microcephaly.
- Chronic encephalitis.
- Cardiac defects.

ENTEROCOCCUS

Enterococcus (*E. faecium, E. casseliflavus, E. faecalis*) colonization in neonates can occur during birth or after birth, often evident on culture within the first day of life. Enterococcus is found in maternal vaginal and gastrointestinal secretions and in human milk. Enterococcus is part of the normal flora, and most colonization is asymptomatic, but in some cases, *Enterococcus* can cause severe neonatal infections. Risk factors for enterococcal infection include low birth rate and preterm birth. In many cases, enterococcus infections are vancomycin-resistant, especially associated with prepartal antibiotic therapy. Infection rates appear to be seasonal with increases in the winter/spring months. About 5% of infants colonized with *Enterococcus* develop necrotizing enterocolitis. Sepsis with *Enterococcus* can result in ventriculitis, endocarditis, and/or meningitis.

ESCHERICHIA COLI AND STAPHYLOCOCCUS AUREUS

Escherichia coli (*E. coli*) is a Gram-negative bacillus and is the predominant bacteria found in human feces. Within the bowel, most *E. coli* serve beneficial purposes; however, some types of *E.coli* pose a risk to neonates. *E. coli* can cause severe neonatal infections, resulting in urinary tract infection, bacteremia, sepsis, and meningitis. The infection may be acquired during or after birth, especially in preterm infants or those who poor immune systems. The most common source of infection is the maternal gastrointestinal tract. Symptoms in the neonate may vary depending upon the site and extent of infection but include poor feeding, diarrhea, fussiness, and fever.

Staphylococcus aureus may occur in the neonate as a hospital-acquired or community-acquired infection and may present with local infection (such as about the catheter insertion site), cellulitis, urinary infection, or systemic infection. Increasingly, infections are methicillin resistant and require second-line antibiotics. Recurrent infection is common with community-acquired *Staph.*

NEONATAL INFECTIONS CAUSED BY MATERNAL STDS

Maternal **sexually-transmitted diseases** can cause infection in the neonate. Common STDs include:

- **Chlamydia**: Infants most commonly exhibit conjunctivitis.
- **Gonorrhea**: Infants exposed to *Neisseria gonorrhoeae* during vaginal delivery most commonly develop bilateral conjunctivitis (ophthalmia neonatorum) if left untreated. In some cases, disseminated gonococcal infection (DGI) can occur in infants.

- **Syphilis**: Infants may be asymptomatic, even with full system infection. Multiple system disorders and abnormalities can occur, including non-viral hepatitis with jaundice, hepatosplenomegaly, pseudoparalysis, pneumonitis, bone marrow failure, myocarditis, meningitis, anemia, edema associated with nephritic syndrome, and a rash on the palms of the hands and soles of the feet
- **Herpes**: Localized lesions may occur at 10-12 days. Disseminated infection may cause pneumonitis, hepatitis, and encephalitis.
- **HIV/AIDS:** Infants are asymptomatic at birth and may test falsely positive.
- **Trichomoniasis**: Infants may be born preterm and with low birth weight (<2500 g).

CHLAMYDIA

Chlamydia is the most common sexually transmitted disease in the United States and can be passed on at the time of birth if the infant is delivered vaginally and comes into contact with contaminated vaginal secretions. The organism responsible for this infection is *Chlamydia trachomatis.* Because the mother infected with this organism is usually asymptomatic, preventive care for the newborn is essential. The usual infection site for the newborn is the eye, in the form of conjunctivitis. States now require all newborns be given a prophylactic dose of either erythromycin or tetracycline ointment in the eyes at birth to prevent this infection. While the antibiotic ointment stops the eye infection, a few infants exposed to the pathogen will develop pneumonitis and/or ear infection.

NEISSERIA GONORRHOEA

Neisseria gonorrhoeae infections are common and may result in recurrent infection, pelvic inflammatory disease (PID), chronic pain, and infertility. Women who become pregnant and have a history of gonorrhea with salpingitis are 7 to 10 times more likely to have an ectopic pregnancy. Signs of infection (dysuria and green foul-smelling discharge from the urethra and the vagina) may occur 3 to 5 days after contact. However, many women are asymptomatic, especially on initial infection, and may be unaware they have the infection while pregnant. Vaginal delivery increases risk to the neonate, but infection can occur with caesarean. Newborns usually develop conjunctivitis 2 to 5 days after birth. Infants exhibit bilateral purulent ocular discharge, edema of the eyelids, and chemosis (edema of conjunctiva). Without treatment, the infection can progress and may result in rupture of the globe and blindness. In rare cases, the neonate may develop sepsis or meningitis from untreated infection. However, routine prophylaxis (usually erythromycin ointment) to the neonate's eyes is an effective treatment.

SYPHILIS

An infant can be exposed to the **syphilis** organism, *Treponema pallidum,* during gestation and become infected *in utero* starting with the 10th-15th week of gestation. Many infected fetuses abort spontaneously or are stillborn. The infant born infected with syphilis can be asymptomatic at birth or can have a full multi-system infection. An infant who is symptomatic may have non-viral hepatitis with jaundice, hepatosplenomegaly, pseudoparalysis, pneumonitis, bone marrow failure, myocarditis, meningitis, anemia, edema associated with nephritic syndrome, and a rash on the palms of the hands and soles of the feet. Other symptoms, such as interstitial keratitis and dental and facial abnormalities may occur as the child develops. Treatment involves an aggressive regimen of penicillin administration with frequent follow-up until blood tests are negative.

OSTEOMYELITIS

Osteomyelitis is an infection of the bone, usually bacterial. Common causative agents include *Staphylococcus aureus,* Group B *Streptococcus,* and *Kingella kingae* (often associated with respiratory infection). Neonates may be essentially asymptomatic in the early stages and diagnosis is most common >3 weeks. Because of the vascularity of the bones in the neonate, systemic infections can spread easily, and once it has invaded the periosteum, it can travel the length of the bone rather than staying localized at a joint (although joint infection may occur secondary to osteomyelitis) and may rupture through the periosteum and infect muscle tissue. Osteomyelitis may be a complication of septic arthritis. Bone scans are usually not effective for diagnosis < 6 months, but aspirant is examined and cultured. Symptoms include fever, muscular tenderness pseudoparalysis of affected limb. Treatment is with aggressive IV therapy followed by oral antibiotics (similar to septic arthritis). Surgical drainage may be done if joint abscesses occur.

EARLY-ONSET SEPSIS
RISK FACTORS AND CAUSES

Early-onset bacterial sepsis usually occurs in the first 24 hours after birth, but may occur any time up to day 6 of life. Infants born prematurely have an increased rate of early-onset sepsis and more rapid onset of symptoms. In early onset sepsis, the source of infection is from the mother, either transplacentally, or a microorganism that colonized the mother's birth canal. Pathogens that most commonly cause early-onset sepsis are Group B Streptococcus, *E. coli*, *Haemophilus influenzae*, coagulase negative *Staphylococcus*, and *Listeria monocytogenes*. Risk factors for the development of early onset sepsis include:

- Premature, preterm, or prolonged rupture of membranes.
- Maternal colonization with Group B *Streptococcus*.
- Fever in the mother greater than 38°C during delivery.
- Premature birth or low birth weight (<2500 g).
- Maternal urinary tract infection.
- Chorioamnionitis.
- APGAR score less than 6 at 1 or 5 minutes.
- Delivery with birth asphyxia or meconium staining.

CLINICAL MANIFESTATIONS AND DIAGNOSIS

The clinical manifestations for **early-onset sepsis** are often vague and nonspecific making it a particular challenge to diagnose early. Sometimes the only noticeable sign is that the mother or nurse will note that the infant just doesn't seem well—nothing that can be specified but just general symptoms perhaps starting with a poor feeding or other seemingly minor event. Infection may localize or cause bacteremia and sometimes meningitis. Some manifestations that should be noted include:

- The inability of the infant to maintain a normal body temperature.
- Apnea, tachypnea.
- Vomiting.
- Cyanosis.
- Lethargy.
- Jaundice.
- Seizures.
- Purpura.

If sepsis is suspected, CSF examination is done to evaluate for possible meningitis, a frequent complication of sepsis, especially if the infant is exhibiting symptoms of sepsis, GBS sepsis, or late onset of infection.

LATE-ONSET SEPSIS

Late-onset sepsis occurs after day 6 of life and is more common in preterm infants and those with medical or surgical conditions. The infection is acquired from the environment after birth, rather than from the mother. Infants with indwelling catheters, nasal cannulae, continuous positive airway pressure (CPAP), intubation, ventricular taps, and any other type of prolonged instrumentation are at increased risk. Late onset sepsis generally has a more gradual onset than early onset sepsis, and the site of primary infection relates to the cause. For example, ventilation-associated infection results in pneumonia. Likely organisms involved in late onset sepsis include:

- Gram-positive organisms like *Staphylococcus aureus* and Group B *Streptococcus* in 2/3 of cases.
- Gram-negative organisms such as *E coli*, *Klebsiella pneumoniae*, P*seudomonas aeruginosa*, Serratia, Enterobacter, and Acinetobacter.
- Candida.

BACTERIAL MENINGITIS

CAUSES AND DISEASE PROCESSES

Bacterial meningitis is caused by a wide range of pathogenic organisms, varying with infant's age:

- ≤1 month; E.coli, Group B Streptococci, Listeria monocytogenes, and Neisseria meningitidis.
- 1-2 months: Group B *Streptococci*.

Bacterial infections usually arise from spread of distant infections but can enter the CNS from surgical wounds, invasive devices, or nasal colonization. The infective process includes inflammation, exudates, white blood cell accumulation, and tissue damage with the brain showing evidence of hyperemia and edema. Purulent exudate covers the brain and invades and blocks the ventricles, obstructing CSF and leading to increased intracranial pressure. Since antibodies specific to bacteria don't cross the blood/brain barrier, the body's ability to fight the infection is very poor.

DIAGNOSIS

Diagnosis is based on examination of cerebrospinal fluid and symptoms. *Symptoms* may be very non-specific, such as hypo- or hyperthermia, jaundice, irritability, lethargy, irregular respirations with periods of apnea, difficulty feeding with loss of suck reflex, hypotonia, weak cry, seizures, and bulging fontanels (late sign). Nuchal rigidity does not usually occur with neonates. Meningitis is often difficult to diagnose in the neonate because it has early nonspecific clinical findings of irritability, lethargy, poor feeding, temperature instability, and hypotension. The more specific neurological symptoms of seizures or bulging fontanels are seen in late onset infection. Antibiotics given to the mother prior to delivery or to the neonate prior to performing a lumbar puncture inhibit bacterial growth in cerebrospinal fluid (CSF), making the diagnosis dependent on other CSF parameters. **CSF findings** suggestive of bacterial meningitis include:

- Decreased glucose.
- Elevated protein.
- White blood cells values in CSR greater than 100 WBC/dL.

A polymerase chain reaction assay test for Group B strep antigen in CSF is available. Values may be more difficult to interpret in the premature neonate, as their blood brain barrier is more permeable.

TREATMENT OF SEPSIS/MENINGITIS

Neonatal sepsis and meningitis are treated with intravenous antibiotics. Usually if sepsis is suspected, treatment with broad-spectrum antibiotics (IV aminoglycoside and penicillin) will be started while awaiting the culture results. Once culture results are obtained any adjustment to a more effective medication to treat the now identified organism may be made. Using antibiotics too liberally when not indicated by a confirmed bacterial infection can have serious consequences for the neonate, such as the development of antibiotic resistant strains of bacteria and the killing of the normal flora of organisms that inhabit the intestinal tract leading to digestive problems. These problems must be weighed with the need to quickly treat a suspected sepsis when cultures have not been completed as many of these take days to finish growing. If hydrocephalus occurs with meningitis, then a ventroperitoneal shunt may be inserted surgically. Enteral or parenteral feedings may be necessary to provide adequate nutrition during treatment. Radiant warmers or incubators may be needed for thermoregulation.

RANGE OF SEVERE INFECTIONS

There are a number of terms used to refer to the **range of severe infections** and often used interchangeably, but they are part of a continuum:

- **Bacteremia** is the present of bacteria in the blood but without systemic infection.
- **Septicemia** is a systemic infection caused by pathogens (usually bacteria or fungi) present in the blood.
- **Systemic inflammatory response syndrome** *(SIRS)*, a generalized inflammatory response affecting may organ systems, may be caused by infectious or non-infectious agents, such as trauma, adrenal insufficiency, pulmonary embolism, and drug overdose. If an infectious agent is identified or suspected, SIRS is an aspect of sepsis. Infective agents for infants include a wide range of bacteria and fungi, including *Streptococcus pneumoniae* and *Staphylococcus aureus.* SIRS includes 2 of the following:
  - Elevated (>38 °C) or subnormal rectal temperature (<36 °C).
  - Tachypnea >60 for infants or $PaCO_2$ <32 mm Hg.
  - Tachycardia >160 for infants.
  - Leukocytosis (>12,000) or leukopenia (<4000).
- **Sepsis** is presence of infection either locally or systemically in which there is a generalized life-threatening inflammatory response (SIRS). It includes all the indications for SIRS as well as one of the following:
  - Hypoxemia (<72 mmHg) without pulmonary disease.
  - Elevation in plasma lactate.
  - Decreased urinary output <5 mL/kg/hr for ≥1 hour.
- **Severe sepsis** includes both indications of SIRS and sepsis as well as indications of increasing organ dysfunction with inadequate perfusion and/or hypotension.
- **Septic shock** is a progression from severe sepsis in which refractory hypotension occurs despite treatment. There may be indications of lactic acidosis.
- **Multi-organ dysfunction syndrome** (MODS) is the most common cause of sepsis-related death. Cardiac function becomes depressed, acute respiratory distress syndrome (ARDS) may develop, and renal failure may follow acute tubular necrosis or cortical necrosis. Thrombocytopenia appears in about 30% of those affected and may result in disseminated intravascular coagulation (DIC). Liver damage and bowel necrosis may occur.

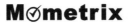

Psychosocial Support, Grieving, and Discharge Planning

DECREASING FAMILY STRESS

Having a neonate admitted to the neonatal intensive care unit is a very stressful event for a family because it interrupts family interactions and the bonding process that occurs when a neonate goes home to spend time with family members. Interventions to decrease **family stress** and encourage bonding between the neonate, mother, and family include:

- Have facilities available for families to stay close to their infant to encourage bonding.
- Maintain a play area for siblings so they are not isolated from parents.
- Permit liberal visiting times for family members.
- If it is known before birth that the infant will require critical care, let the family visit the unit and ask questions.
- Give the family contact information for support groups comprised of other parents who have children with similar illnesses.
- Encourage hands-on parental care, including kangaroo care, by both parents.

SIBLING RESPONSES/INTERVENTIONS

Siblings should be included, and parents are encouraged to bring them to visit and interact, as much as possible, with the neonate. If the neonate has abnormalities, this may cause stress to the siblings. Younger children may be hostile and older children ashamed. They may feel guilty about their responses, and they may feel neglected as parents go through the stages of grief and are unable to provide the support that the siblings need. In some cases, parents may express their concern by focusing their anxiety on one of the siblings, becoming hypercritical. In these cases, staff may need to intervene by discussing observations with the parents and encouraging other family members to provide support to the siblings. Parents' groups that involve the entire family can be very helpful. Whenever possible, children should be included in education and demonstrations and encouraged to ask questions. Age-appropriate books and other materials that explain medical conditions and treatments should be available for siblings.

PREPARATION OF SIBLINGS FOR BIRTH OF INFANT

Preparation of siblings prior to the birth of an infant can decrease anxiety and sibling rivalry by helping the children feel that they are participants in the process and are valued. Children should be prepared for physical changes in the mother, changing family dynamics, and infant care. Formal classes may be available for children ages 3 to 12 to help them identify and express their concerns, and to teach them about pregnancy and childcare. Booklets, books, and videos are also available. The parent/teacher may use dolls to demonstrate childcare and allow the children to practice holding and caring for the baby. When possible, children should have contact with an infant, such as that of a friend or family member. Children may help to decorate the infant's room or prepare a "welcome" gift, such as a drawing or toy. Children should be told who will care for them during labor and delivery and should visit the mother and infant as soon after delivery as possible.

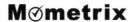

BARRIERS TO PARENT-INFANT INTERACTION

There are many **barriers to parent-infant interaction**, especially with preterm infants or those with genetic disabilities or birth defects that require prolonged hospitalization or treatment. Barriers include:

- **Physical separation:** When the infant cannot be held or fed, when the child is transported to a different facility outside of the area, or when the mother is discharged and the infant remains hospitalized, this prevents attachment.
- **Lack of clear understanding of handicaps and/or developmental problems:** Lack of infant response is sometimes interpreted as rejection, and parents may be frightened by abnormalities.
- **Attitude of medical staff:** Negative attitudes may cause the parent to grieve rather than attach to the child. Staff members need to encourage the parents to become involved in the child's care and to provide stimulation. Staff often needs to demonstrate care to parents, who may be intimidated by the infant's condition and medical needs.
- **Environmental overload:** The equipment (alarms, ventilators, monitors) and environmental constraints (no chairs) may overwhelm parents.

MATERNAL ATTACHMENT PROCESS

By the time of birth, most mothers have developed an emotional connection with their infants and demonstrate a number of typical steps in the **maternal attachment process**.

- **Touching:** The mother usually begins by lightly touching the infant's extremities with her fingertips and running her palm over the baby's trunk. This exploration of the infant can proceed very quickly in minutes, or be more tentative and take days. Early skin-to-skin contact with the infant tends to accelerate this process.
- **En face positioning:** The mother increases the amount of face-to-face eye contact with the infant, typically holding the infant close to her face and responding to eye contact by speaking in a sing-song high-pitched tone (baby talk).
- **Responding:** The mother tends to respond verbally to sounds the infant makes. Initially, the mother may feel separate and distant from the child, especially if she doesn't feel an immediate bond, and she should be reassured that these feelings are normal.

ACQUAINTANCE

During the acquaintance period, the first few days, responding helps the mother to recognize **clues** the child is giving about needs, such as hunger. The mother's ability to respond to those needs strengthens the bond and helps her gain confidence in her parenting ability. During this time, the infant is also learning to recognize **routines**, such as nursing when held toward the breast.

MUTUAL REGULATION

During this phase, which may vary in duration, the mother is learning to **balance** the needs of the infant against her own needs, and she may have some negative feelings, such as resenting her lack of sleep or feeling frustrated by the infant's crying. The mother may be afraid to express any negative feelings, fearful that people will think she is a "bad" mother, but these feelings are normal and are likely to continue until the mother and infant reach a mutual balance. The ability of the mother and infant to recognize each other's cues and respond to them is termed **reciprocity**.

MATERNAL ATTACHMENT/BONDING ASSESSMENT

Assessment of maternal attachment/bonding should be done prior to discharge so that any issues and needed interventions can be discussed. In doing the assessment, the nurse evaluates the mother's

- progression in touching and face-to-face eye contact with extended times and indications of attraction, such as verbally responding to the infant and cuddling the infant. If there has been no progression, the nurse should assess contributing environmental, cultural, and social factors that may be interfering.
- consistency in caring for the infant and seeking knowledge about and validation of her infant care; adjusting care to the needs of the infant. Sensitivity to infant's needs, such as recognizing discomfort or hunger quickly and exhibiting pleasure at infant's response to her efforts.
- pleasure in the infant, expressed by calling the infant by name, noting family traits/characteristics, showing overt happiness. If the mother shows displeasure or apathy, this may indicate poor attachment, but might also indicate that the mother is experiencing pain or weakness.

PATERNAL AND SIBLING/FAMILY BONDING

Paternal attachment, referred to as engrossment, occurs in many ways similar to maternal attachment. The father may feel pride and wonderment at the child and develop a strong sense of nurturing. Early and frequent contact with the infant promotes engrossment, so the nurse should ensure that the father is not overlooked after delivery but is able to hold, touch, and respond to the child as soon as possible.

Sibling and family attachment are important. Siblings should be allowed to visit the mother and infant as early as possible and be encouraged to hold or care for the infant as appropriate for their ages. Siblings sometimes feel left out or overshadowed by the new infant, so it's important that the parents take time to talk to the siblings and give them attention as well. Grandparents and other family members also form attachments to the infant and should be included.

CULTURAL/LIFESTYLE FACTORS AFFECTING FAMILY INTEGRATION

VALUES

Values based on attitudes, ideas, and beliefs often connect family members to common **goals**. However, these values may be influenced by many **external factors**, such as education, social norms, and attitudes of peers, other family, and coworkers, so values may change and this may impact family integration.

ROLES

In some families, roles are clearly defined by **gender** and **task** (homemaker and breadwinner), but the roles blur or are **shared** in many families, and in some cases, the father becomes the primary caregiver while the mother works. Other common roles include peacemaker, nurturer, and social planner. How these roles are perceived and actualized affects the manner in which a child is integrated into the family.

DECISION-MAKING

Family power structures vary widely, but in many families, **power** rests with one person who makes ultimate decisions and whose opinions affect other family members. In cultures with a strong emphasis on tradition, power often lies with the father, a grandparent, or another family member. However, it should not be assumed that families of a given cultural background will always have the same power structure. Instead, power may be **shared** or it may rest with either the mother or the father.

SOCIOECONOMIC

Employment trends, marriage rates, and economic trends all affect **family integration**. Many people have become unemployed and are unable to support their families, resulting in severe **stress**, which may be exacerbated by the arrival of a new child. The divorce rate is high, leaving many parents with inadequate funds to support a child. Even if both parents are employed, the cost of living continues to escalate, including the cost of caring for a child.

FAMILY TYPES

Some of the different types of families are described below:

- **Nuclear** – This **husband-wife-children** model was once the most common family type but is no longer the norm. In this model, the husband is the provider, and the mother stays home to care for the children. This makes up only about **7%** of current American families.
- **Dual career/dual earner** – This model, where **both parents work**, is the most common in American society, affecting about **66%** of two-parent families. One parent may work more than another, or both may work fulltime. There may be disparities in income that affect family dynamics.
- **Childless** – Ten to fifteen percent have no children because of **infertility** or **choice**.
- **Extended** – These may include **multigenerational families** or **shared households** with friends, parents, or other relatives. Childcare responsibilities may be shared or primarily assumed by an extended family member, such as a grandparent.
- **Extended kin network** – Two or more nuclear families live close together, share goods and services, and support each other, including sharing childcare. This model is common in the Hispanic community.

SINGLE-PARENT

This is one of the fastest growing family models. Typically, the mother is the single parent, but in some cases, it is the father. The single parent may be widowed, divorced, or separated, but more commonly, has never married. In cases of divorce or abandonment, the child may have minimal or no contact with one parent, often the father. Single parents often face difficulties in trying to **support and care for a child** and may suffer **economic hardship**.

STEPPARENT

Because of the high rate of divorce, stepparent families are common. This can result in **stress** and **conflict** when a new child enters the picture. There may be jealousy and resentment on the part of siblings and estranged family members. In some cases, families can work together to achieve harmony and provide added support to children.

BINUCLEAR/CO-PARENTING

In this model, children share time between two primarily nuclear families because of **joint custody agreements**. While this may at times result in conflict, the child benefits from having a continued relationship with both parents.

COHABITING

Unmarried heterosexual couples live together. The relationships within this model may vary, with some similar to the nuclear family. In some cases, people are in committed relationships and may avoid marriage because of economic or personal reasons. A planned child may strengthen the relationship, but an unplanned child may cause conflict.

GAY/LESBIAN

Whether gays and lesbians marry or cohabit, they create families in **non-traditional ways**. For example, lesbians may use sperm donors. Gay couples often adopt. Children in these families may face social pressures because of their parents' lifestyles.

MOTHER RELINQUISHING CHILD FOR ADOPTION

A mother relinquishing her child for **adoption** may have feelings of ambivalence and sadness. Many who relinquish their infants for adoption are young and/or unmarried. Adoptions may be closed or open, so procedures will vary. In some open adoptions, the adoptive parent(s) may accompany the mother and participate in the birth, with the birth mother relinquishing the child immediately after birth. In this case, the adoptive parents should be treated as the actual parents of the child, while staff should recognize the needs of the birth mother and provide for her emotional and physical support. In other cases, the child is first relinquished to an agency, such as Social Services, which then places the child. If possible, prior to the birth, the birth mother should indicate how she wants to handle the birth. Some want to hold and spend time with the child; others do not. The birth mother should be in a single room, rather than with other mothers, to protect her privacy.

STAGES OF GRIEF

Grief is a normal response to the death or severe illness/abnormality of an infant or fetus. How a person deals with grief is very personal, and each person will grieve differently. Elisabeth Kubler-Ross identified **five stages of grief** in *On Death and Dying* (1969). A person may not go through each stage but usually goes through two of the five stages:

- **Denial**: The parents may be resistive to information and unable to accept that a child is dying/impaired or believe that the child is not theirs. They may act stunned, immobile, or detached and may be unable to respond appropriately or remember what's said, often repeatedly asking the same questions.
- **Anger**: As reality becomes clear, parents may react with pronounced anger, directed inward or outward. Women, especially, may blame themselves and self-anger may lead to severe depression and guilt, assuming they are to blame because of some action before or during pregnancy. Outward anger, more common in men, may be expressed as overt hostility. (Continued)
- **Bargaining**: This involves if-then thinking (often directed at a deity): "If I go to church every way, then God will prevent this." Parents may change doctors, trying to change the outcome.
- **Depression**: As the parents begin to accept the loss, they may become depressed, feeling no one understands and overwhelmed with sadness. They may be tearful or crying and may withdraw or ask to be left alone.
- **Acceptance**: This final stage represents a form of resolution and often occurs outside of the medical environment after months. Parents are able to resume their normal activities and lose the constant preoccupation with their child. They are able to think of the child without severe pain. With a disabled child, acceptance may be delayed because of daily challenges and reminders.

TYPES OF GRIEF

Anticipatory grief occurs when a child is diagnosed with a terminal illness. The parent begins to mourn over the loss of the child before he or she expires.

Incongruent grief occurs when the mother and the father are "out of synch" in their grieving process, stressing their relationship. It may be due to the differences in how men and women grieve, or it may be because the woman typically bonds with the infant during the pregnancy, while the father bonds after the child is born.

Delayed grief occurs when the grieving process is postponed months to years after the loss of a child. Initially, the parent may not be able to grieve appropriately, because of an inability to cope, or the pressing need to care for other family members.

GENDER DIFFERENCES IN GRIEVING

When faced with the death of a child, **men and women** generally grieve differently:

- **Women** are often more expressive about their loss and more emotional. They are more likely to look for support from others. **Men** often grieve in a more solitary and cognitive manner. They are generally more oriented to fact-gathering or problem-solving.
- The bond that develops between a pregnant woman and the developing fetus is unique and generally very intense. The father often forms a stronger bond after the birth of the child.

When one parent does not grieve in the same fashion as the other (**incongruent grieving**) this may be a source of conflict in their marriage. How a person acts on the outside is not always a true indicator of how that person is feeling on the inside.

FACTORS THAT INFLUENCE GRIEVING FAMILIES

The emotions that individuals and families experience with the loss or severe illness/disability of an infant are varied and dependent on many factors that influence grief:

- **Cultural influences**: Different cultures have their own practices and beliefs concerning sickness, death, and dying, and varying rituals and ceremonies for processing loss.
- **Family system**: The family's composition, the roles of its various members, and its economic circumstances affect its expression of grief. A large family with extended community support processes grief differently from a single mother living far from home.
- **Siblings**: The impact on other children in the family must be considered, in addition to the impact on the parents.
- **History of loss**: Many diseases have a genetic component, and this may not be the first child to be affected.

Review Video: Patient Treatment and Grief
Visit mometrix.com/academy and enter code: 648794

Review Video: Coping with a Disability
Visit mometrix.com/academy and enter code: 630500

INTERVENTIONS FOR CIRCUMSTANCES THAT LEAD TO GRIEF

Parents may need extra support in **circumstances that lead to grief**:

- **Chronic sorrow**: If grief is prolonged and the individual does not seem to be able to move forward, the individual should be encouraged to talk about feelings and express grief openly and to seek outside support, such as a therapist or support group.
- **Death of a twin, triplet, or other multiple**: The parents should be encouraged to name the child and allowed to hold the child if possible and to talk about the child and express feelings of loss. Some parents may want to keep a tangible memory, such as a clipping of hair or a hand- or footprint of the child. Some may benefit from a support group.
- **Repeated obstetric loss** (recurrent abortion, still birth, preterm delivery): The losses should be acknowledged by those caring for the parents ("I'm so sorry....") and the parents encouraged to express feeling about their loss.

DISCHARGE REQUIREMENTS

In the past, **discharge requirements** included weight or post conceptual weight requirements. Current requirements are instead based on physiological and functional readiness. Hospitals vary, but requirements generally include:

- All medical or surgical problems that require hospitalization are resolved.
- The infant is feeding appropriately, as evidenced by:
  - Primary caregiver feeding the infant with the prescribed method (gavage, gastrostomy, or special positioning).
  - Weight gain of 15-30 grams per day over several days.
  - Feeds accomplished without respiratory difficulty.
- Temperature stability is maintained in an open crib.
- Parents are trained appropriately concerning administration of medications, CPR, and proper use of car seat.
- Infant has passed all pre-discharge tests:
  - Hearing screening.
  - Other tests as needed (anemia, ROP exams, sleep study, head ultrasound).
- Age appropriate immunizations were administered.
- Discharge environment has been evaluated.
- Appropriate post discharge follow-up appointments are scheduled with specialists and the primary care physician.

FOLLOW-UP SCREENING FROM NEONATE TO CHILDHOOD

Many **screening procedures** are available; including extensive laboratory testing that may be indicated if there is cause for concern that an infant may have a disorder. However, some basic screening should be done for all infants and children:

- **Genetic disorders:** Screening is usually done at birth according to state guidelines, and then may be indicated if there is concern that a child has a disorder that requires treatment.
- **Hearing:** Testing is usually done with newborns and then every 2-3 years until age 18.
- **Height and weight:** These are monitored monthly during the first year and then at least yearly until age 18 to determine if the child's development is within the normal range.
- **Vision:** This is screened at birth, at 3-4 years, and periodically between 5-18. Vision problems may become obvious when the child enters school and can't see the board or has trouble reading.
- **Fasting blood sugar:** Done every 2 years for those at risk. (Continued)
- **Head circumference:** Measurement is done at birth, 1 year, and 2 years.
- **Blood pressure:** This is usually checked during infancy (6-12 months) and then periodically throughout childhood.
- **Dental screening:** Bottle fed babies may require earlier screening as they often fall asleep with the bottle in their mouths, leading to infant caries. Dental screening is done periodically throughout childhood, especially after the new teeth come in to evaluate for malocclusion or other problems.
- **Alcohol/drug use:** Neonates are screened for parental abuse. Screening of use may be done periodically for children between 11-18 years, especially if they are at risk.
- **Developmental screening:** There are a number of screening tests that are available and can be used if a child appears to have a developmental delay or abnormality. Screening tests must be age-appropriate. The tests are not diagnostic, but can help to confirm developmental abnormalities. Tests may assess motor skills, language, and cognitive ability.

UNIVERSAL HEARING SCREENING PRIOR TO DISCHARGE

Universal hearing screening is recommended by the AAP for all newborns. Hearing loss in neonates may occur because of genetic abnormalities, *in utero* infections with cytomegalovirus or rubella, meningitis, craniofacial abnormalities, or Usher's syndrome. Admission to the NICU for longer than two days increases the likelihood of hearing loss by tenfold, so all newborns should be screened for hearing loss — not just those with risk factors — prior to discharge. Undiagnosed hearing loss results in severe language and developmental delay. Identification and early intervention during the critical time period of language development decreases the morbidity associated with neonatal hearing loss. Reasons for screening include:

- An easy-to-use test is available with high degrees of sensitivity and specificity.
- Hearing loss is otherwise difficult to detect until language milestones have been missed
- Interventions are available to correct conditions.
- Early intervention results in improved outcome.
- The screening process can be performed in a cost-effective manner.

PRINCIPLES OF ADULT LEARNING

Adults have a wealth of life and/or employment experiences. Their attitudes toward education may vary considerably. There are, however, some **principles of adult learning** and typical characteristics of adult learners that an instructor should consider when planning strategies for teaching patients and families.

Practical/Goal-Oriented	Provide overviews or summaries and examples.
	Use collaborative discussions with problem-solving exercises.
	Remain organized with the goal in mind.
Self-Directed	Provide active involvement, asking for input.
	Allow different options toward achieving the goal.
	Give responsibilities.
Knowledgeable	Show respect for life experiences/ education.
	Validate knowledge and ask for feedback.
	Relate new material to information with which they are familiar.
Relevancy-Oriented	Explain how information will be applied.
	Clearly identify objectives.
Motivated	Provide certificates of achievement, if possible, or other tangible reward.

VISUAL-AUDITORY-KINESTHETIC MODEL OF COGNITIVE LEARNING

Not all people are aware of their preferred **learning style.** A range of teaching materials and methods that relates to all 3 learning preferences—visual, auditory, kinesthetic—and are appropriate for different ages and should be available. Part of assessment for teaching involves choosing the right approach, based on observation and feedback. Presenting learners with different options often gives a clue to their preferred learning style. Some people have a combined learning style.

Visual learners learn best by seeing and reading.	Provide written directions, picture guides, or demonstrate procedures.
	Use charts and diagrams.
	Provide photos, videos.
Auditory learners learn best by listening and talking.	Plan extra time to discuss and answer questions.
	Provide audiotapes.
	Explain procedures while demonstrating and have learner repeat.
Kinesthetic learners learn best by handling, doing, and practicing.	Provide hands-on experience throughout teaching.
	Encourage handling of supplies/equipment.
	Allow learner to demonstrate.
	Minimize instructions and allow person to explore equipment and procedures.

READABILITY

Studies have indicated that learning is more effective if oral presentations and/or demonstrations are supplemented with reading materials, such as handouts. **Readability** (the grade level of material) is a concern because many patients and families may have limited English skills or low literacy, and it can be difficult for the nurse to assess people's reading level. The average American reads effectively at the sixth to eighth grade level, regardless of education achieved, but many health education materials are written at a much higher level. Additionally, research indicates that even people with much higher reading skills learn medical and health information most effectively when the material is presented at the sixth to eighth grade level. Therefore, patient education materials and consent forms should not be written at higher than the sixth to eighth grade level. Readability index calculators are available on the Internet to assist in preparing materials by giving an approximation of grade level and difficulty for those without expertise in teaching reading.

EDUCATIONAL NEEDS OF NEW MOTHERS

The **educational needs** of the new mother and family vary depending on age, background, education, experience, and expectations. The needs of the adolescent mother with no experience may be quite different from those of the multiparous mother. Assessing individual needs can be difficult in the short time women are usually hospitalized, so education should cover a wide range of topics. A checklist of topics may be a helpful starting point for the mother to indicate her needs. Because mothers are usually fatigued for the first 24 to 48 hours, teaching after that time is most effective, but many mothers leave the hospital on the second day. Demonstration with return demonstration is an effective method to ensure that a mother can carry out tasks, but education should anticipate other needs and concerns that may arise. Mothers often have concerns about a variety of issues, such as childcare, contraception, and resuming sexual relations. Pamphlets, website information, or videos that can be sent home with the mother are very helpful.

NEWBORN CARE FOR SPECIAL-NEEDS NEONATES

Family involvement and education are vital for successful discharge of a **special-needs neonate** to ensure proper care. Bringing home a premature infant or one who has special needs is a daunting task for any parent, so preparation is essential.

- Educate the parents or guardians about appropriate care methods.
- Explain how to interpret the infant's cues concerning his needs and how to respond appropriately.
- Point out the different states of alertness during their infant's sleep and wake cycles. Identify the appropriate times and methods for infant interaction.
- Coach the parents to ensure that they perform each skill correctly and retain it. Observe interaction between the infant and parents in the nursery to help ensure continued wellness of the infant after discharge.
- Encourage kangaroo care immediately after birth for stable newborns as it is an excellent method to foster bonding between the neonate and the mother. For neonates who require resuscitation and medical intervention, delay kangaroo care until the neonate is stable.
- If the parents are not ready, contact a social worker for follow-up.

ANTICIPATORY GUIDANCE FOR INFANT WITH CONGENITAL RUBELLA SYNDROME

Infants who have been diagnosed as having **congenital rubella syndrome** will secrete this active virus in their urine and stool for many years after birth. This requires that parents be extensively taught about the risk their infant could pose to pregnant women who are not immune to rubella or who do not know their status. The mother of an infant with this disorder should have a titer drawn to ensure that they are shown as immune so as to prevent future pregnancies from being affected. The parents need to be taught that they have a responsibility to protect others from exposure but to make sure that in the process they are not treating the infant in such a way so as to completely isolate him from the outside world.

ANTICIPATORY GUIDANCE FOR INFANT REQUIRING HOME CARDIORESPIRATORY MONITORS

Some infants may be discharged on **cardiorespiratory monitors**. These monitors have been shown to be successful in preventing death from apnea for certain infants. These monitors are NOT indicated for the prevention of SIDS in an otherwise healthy newborn. The following events are indications that an infant may be sent home on monitors:

- Infant who has apnea of prematurity that has had all other causes of apnea ruled out.
- Infant who survived an apparent life-threatening event (ALTE) and that event was apnea, cyanosis, choking or gagging.
- Infant who has had two or more siblings who have died from SIDS
- Infant with a tracheostomy.

Parents/caregivers must have a clear understanding of the reasons for the monitors and how to apply, remove, and care for them. They should have hospital practice and should demonstrate their skills before discharge of the infants.

ANTICIPATORY GUIDANCE FOR INFANT EXPOSED TO SUBSTANCES OF ABUSE *IN UTERO*

Infants exposed to perinatal drugs of abuse require a multidisciplinary team approach when preparing for discharge. These high-risk infants may still be dealing with physical withdrawal symptoms. They have possible developmental delays. They may return to a toxic home (marijuana grow-op, methamphetamine lab, crack house, or bordello). Ensure that:

- A case manager is assigned to all infants to coordinate the discharge process.
- Postpartum length of stay is flexible, as the infant may not display symptoms of withdrawal until 7 days of age.
- The mother is allowed to room-in to facilitate special teaching concerning withdrawal symptoms and to strengthen the infant-maternal bonding process.
- A public health nurse or protective social worker is scheduled to perform a home evaluation within one week of discharge.
- Mothers (and fathers) who are not already enrolled in a drug abuse treatment program are referred to an appropriate program.

ANTICIPATORY GUIDANCE FOR INFANT WITH CARDIAC DISORDER

Parents caring for an **infant with a cardiac disorder** should be taught to call the physician if their infants exhibit any of the following symptoms:

- Poor feeding that lasts more than a couple of days.
- Sweating or grunting while feeding (any signs that feeding is extra work or tiring them out).
- Vomiting the majority of what is eaten in a 12-24 hour period of time.
- Breathing that is faster than normal or that looks or sounds labored and lasts for several hours.
- A significant and noticeable decrease in the activity level of the infant.
- Any weight loss or failure to gain weight for a significant period of time.
- A change in skin or perioral color (cyanosis).
- A higher than normal incidence of respiratory type illnesses (cold, croup, etc.).

These instructions should be written down for the parents to take home and refer to, as one cannot rely on the memory of already stressed parents for something this important.

EDUCATION REGARDING FECAL ELIMINATION

The first stool (**meconium**) is usually passed within 48 hours and is black and tarry looking. The stool then transitions to greenish as the baby nurses or takes formula, and by the third day, the stool is usually yellow or yellow-green for breastfed babies and yellow or light brown for formula-fed babies. Typically, babies have 2 to 3 stools daily by day 3 and ≥4 daily by day 5, but this may vary:

- Report abnormalities, such as bloody stools, watery stools, very hard stools, clay-colored or whitish stools, black stools (after meconium has passed), and "currant jelly" stools.
- Cleanse skin thoroughly after defecation with mild soap and water, plain water, or unscented baby wipes.
- Examine skin carefully for irritation.

EDUCATION REGARDING URINARY ELIMINATION AND CRADLE CAP

URINARY ELIMINATION

Urination is estimated according to the number of **wet diapers** in a 24-hour period. Typically, the infant has 1 wet diaper the first day, 2 the next, and so on until urination stabilizes at 6 to 8 wet diapers by about day 6.

- Check diaper frequently. Infants often urinate during or after feeding.
- Change diapers when wet, gently cleansing skin with mild soap and water, plain water, or unscented baby wipes.

CRADLE CAP

Cradle cap may appear as scaly, crusted, or flaky skin on the scalp and other parts of the face. It is not contagious and usually clears by 1 or 2 months. It is not usually a sign of poor hygiene.

- Cleanse scalp or affected areas thoroughly, gently rubbing with a terry cloth or brushing with fingers to loosen crust or flakes.
- If persistent, try softening the crusts with olive oil, wait 15 minutes, and then brush or gently comb to loosen crusts or flakes. Finally, wash with baby shampoo.

EDUCATION REGARDING DIAPER RASH

Diaper rash usually results from leaving the infant in soiled/wet diapers and/or not adequately cleansing the skin, although breastfed infants sometimes react to foods the mother has eaten. A rash may also indicate an allergic response to baby wipes or other products, such as lotions or creams. Antibiotics may cause diaper rash. In some cases, a **fungal infection** may occur, usually characterized by red, weepy open areas. Purulent discharge may indicate infection.

- Change diapers as soon as possible when wet or soiled.
- Cleanse skin gently with water.
- Remove diaper and expose the skin to air whenever possible.
- Apply barrier cream or ointment especially formulated for diaper rash to prevent or treat diaper rash.
- Contact physician if rash worsens and does not respond to treatment, as antifungals, cortisone, or topical antibiotics may be indicated.

EDUCATION FOR BREASTFEEDING

Neonates should be fed on demand. Most newborns nurse every 2 to 3 hours or bottle-feed every 2 to 4 hours (8 to 12 times daily) for 20 to 40 minutes. Over time, the infant will establish a more regular feeding schedule, but this may vary widely.

- Try to recognize clues that the infant is hungry and nurse/feed before the infant begins crying frantically. Signs of hunger include licking, rooting, sucking, making fists, bringing hands to mouth, and bobbing the head.
- If you stroke the infant's cheek or lower lip, a hungry infant will usually turn and try to suck the finger.
- Monitor the number of diapers and stools per day, as decrease to less than the average number may indicate dehydration and inadequate nursing/feeding.
- Observe the infant's behavior closely, as some infants nurse for a while and then nap at the breast or take a break before resuming nursing/feeding. A full baby often turns away from the breast/bottle, stops sucking, or resists feeding.

EDUCATION REGARDING CHOKING OR GAGGING

Education regarding chocking/gagging should include the following:

- Ensure small hazardous items, such as pins and cotton balls or materials, such as baby powder are out of reach.
- DO NOT prop bottle for feeding.
- Burp infant regularly during feedings, whether breast or bottle.
- Keep baby in upright position with head elevated during feedings.
- Check nipple of bottle to ensure it is dripping and not running freely.
- If infant is choking, secure face down on forearm, tilted downward, and use the heel of the hand to thump in the mid-back. Repeat as necessary. If choking does not resolve with evidence of breathing immediately, call 911 and begin CPR.

Note: Prevention is important, as most **choking and gagging episodes** can be avoided.

EDUCATION REGARDING BURPING

Both breastfed and bottle-fed babies require **burping** because they swallow air when feeding, although bottle-fed babies tend to require more burping. Infants often show indications (grimacing, squirming, spitting up, and crying) that they are uncomfortable and need to burp.

- Burp the infant routinely after 2 or 3 ounces of formula or after nursing on one breast.
- Position the infant on the shoulder with a burp cloth under the infant's head and gently pat or rub the infant's back.
- Change to a different position if the baby doesn't burp. Try on the opposite shoulder or with the infant sitting on the lap supported by one hand while the other hand pats or rubs the infant's back.

EDUCATION REGARDING CIRCUMCISION

Circumcision rates have dropped by 10% over the last 30 years, with about 58% of male infants now being **circumcised** in the United States. The American Academy of Pediatrics has confirmed that the benefits outweigh the risks, though they do not have a formal recommendation for circumcision and instead leave that decision up to the parents. Benefits including decreased risk of prostate cancer, urinary tract infections, and sexually transmitted diseases such as HIV. Most parents make their decision based on cultural or religious beliefs or the factor of cost, as some insurance companies and many Medicaid programs do not cover the cost of circumcision. While at one time infants were not thought to experience pain, it is now clear that they do, so circumcision should be done using a local anesthesia or topical EMLA cream. After circumcision, the end of the foreskin is typically swollen and red, and some small amount of bleeding may persist for 24 hours. Change the diaper immediately, because urine may cause pain to the open tissue. Cleanse the area gently with water and pat dry. Apply petroleum jelly gauze to the incision area as directed by the individual physician. Avoid using soap or commercial cleansing products, such as baby wipes, until the circumcision heals. Report any change, such as increased swelling, redness, temperature, or purulent discharge.

EDUCATION REGARDING THE UNCIRCUMCISED PENIS AND FONTANELS

UNCIRCUMCISED PENIS

The infant's foreskin is different from the adult male's and does not **separate and retract** until the child is ≥5 years old.

- DO NOT attempt to retract the foreskin.
- DO NOT use cotton swabs to clean.
- Wash the penis with soap and water or just water during the routine bath.

FONTANELS

The infant's fontanels (anterior and posterior) are covered by thick membranous tissue and should feel flat but firm.

- DO NOT be afraid to touch the fontanels or cleanse the scalp.
- Report **bulging** above the level of the skull, as this may indicate increased intracranial pressure.
- Report a **soft fontanel** that sinks below the level of the skull, as this may indicate dehydration.

EDUCATION REGARDING UMBILICAL CORD CARE

Education surrounding the **umbilical cord** should include the following information:

- Protect the cord from moisture, with top of diaper folded under the cord instead of covering it.
- If the cord becomes soiled, wash with mild soap and water, rinse, and dry. Swabbing with alcohol is no longer recommended and may increase skin irritation.
- Avoid covering the cord stump with clothing, which may cause irritation.
- Give the infant only sponge baths until the cord falls off in about 10 to 14 days.
- Report signs of infection, such as erythema, swelling, or purulent discharge.

Note: The umbilical cord changes color from grayish-brown to black as it dries and finally falls off.

EDUCATION REGARDING BATHS

The infant should receive **sponge baths** until the cord falls off at 10 to14 days, and then a bath in an **infant tub** (NOT in an adult tub). Mild soap/shampoo intended for babies or water alone may be used for the bath.

- Make sure the environmental temperature is warm.
- Fill tub with 2 to 3 inches of water.
- ALWAYS check water temperature to make sure it is warm and *not hot*.

- Set hot water heaters ≤120 °F to prevent inadvertent scalding.
- Support the baby during the bath with one arm under upper back to support the neck and head while holding the infant under the axillae.
- Pour water over the child with the free hand and use that hand to wash the hair and the body.
- Lift the baby from the tub and wrap in a towel to dry.
- Dry thoroughly, making sure all skin folds and crevices are dry to prevent irritation and rashes.
- Avoid use of lotions or creams.

EDUCATION REGARDING SAFE POSITIONING OF INFANT

Infants should be placed on their **backs** for sleeping. Sleeping on the stomach increases the risk of **sudden infant death syndrome (SIDS)**.

- Position the infant on the back when unattended or sleeping, but alternate the direction the head faces to prevent one side of the head from flattening (**positional molding**).
- Provide supervised time each day with the infant lying on the abdomen (only on firm surfaces) to strengthen head and neck muscles and to prevent positional molding.
- Hold the infant, rather than leaving them in a carrier.
- Position baby in side-lying position, alternating from one side to the other, using specially designed supports to maintain the position.

EDUCATION REGARDING INFANT CAR SEAT

All infants, regardless of age, must be placed properly in an **infant car seat** during transit. Holding an infant while the car is in motion is not safe. Car seats should be new or in very good condition and fastened according to the manufacturer's guidelines to ensure safety.

- Place the car seat in the back seat and from any side airbags.
- Always securely buckle the child into the seat.
- Face the infant seat toward the rear of the car.
- Recline the seat so the infant's head does not fall forward.
- Place padding around (not under) the infant if the infant slouches to one side.
- Place blankets over the straps and buckles, not under.

ELEMENTS OF DISCHARGE TEACHING

PLAGIOCEPHALY AND FEEDING

Plagiocephaly is an abnormal shape of the head, such as a flat head from lying in the supine position most of the time. With back sleeping, the parents must be aware of the need to place the neonate on the abdomen when awake and supervised. Premature neonates are at increased risk, especially if they spend extended periods on a respirator with head in midline position. Some neonates may have torticollis of neck muscles, causing the head to tilt to one side. This muscle shortening may also occur if the caregiver always holds or feeds the child in the same position. Treatment includes changing positions and sometimes wearing a helmet.

Feeding varies depending on whether the neonate is breastfed or bottle fed, but parents should understand the signs of hunger, correct feeding procedures, and the usual frequency and amounts of feeding necessary for the neonate and older neonates. Initially, neonates nurse every 1 to 3 hours (8 to 12 times/24 hours). Newborns should nurse or bottle feed at least every 3 hours until the birth weight has been regained.

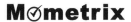

SHAKEN BABY SYNDROME AND CCHD SCREENING

Shaken baby syndrome is believed to be the result of vigorous shaking of a neonate, causing acute subdural hematoma with subarachnoid, and retinal hemorrhages. The shaking of the brain may damage vessels and nerves with resultant cerebral edema. Parents should be advised of the importance of always supporting and protecting the neonate's head and avoiding activities that many injure the child, such as throwing and catching a neonate or small child. Parents should be advised that sometimes children may not exhibit obvious neurological symptoms immediately after trauma but have learning disabilities and behavioral disorders that appear in school.

Critical congenital heart defect (CCHD) screening should be done for all neonates, at time of discharge or ≥24 hours, to identify heart defects as early as possible. Testing is carried out noninvasively with a pulse oximeter to measure oxygen saturation. An initial screen is carried out and may be repeated in one hour and again in 2 hours if results are subpar. A passed screening should show consistent SpO_2 of ≥95% in right hand and foot with ≤3% difference between the two.

RSV

Respiratory syncytial virus (RSV) is a common cause of respiratory illness in infants, especially bronchiolitis and pneumonia. RSV is especially a concern from November to April and is transmitted through droplets spread through coughing and sneezing. Neonates are most at risk for serious illness, especially preterm or ill neonates. Indications of infection include apnea, cough, wheezing, hypoxemia, hypercapnia, and general respiratory distress leading to respiratory failure. The neonate may feed poorly and appear lethargic and irritable. Diagnosis is per rapid viral antigen detection. Treatment depends on the severity of symptoms but may include oxygen, IV fluids, and assisted ventilation. RSV specific treatment and/or prophylaxis includes:

- Palivizumab (Synagis®): Humanized monoclonal antibody (not technically a vaccine) indicated to treat or protect against respiratory syncytial virus for neonates with severe respiratory disease, such as bronchopulmonary dysplasia. Synagis is also recommended for high risk infants with cardiopulmonary disorders, premature infants (≤35 weeks), or those <6 months during the beginning of RSV season. Given monthly for 5 months. Dosage is 15 mg/kg IM.

Adverse effects may include local irritation, diarrhea, vomiting, sore throat, rhinorrhea, rash, pruritis, urticaria, and dyspnea.

Professional Issues

Ethical Principles

AUTONOMY AND JUSTICE

Autonomy is the ethical principle that the individual has the right to make decisions about his/her own care. In the case of neonates, the infant cannot make autonomous decisions, so the parents serve as the legal decision maker. The nurse must keep the parents fully informed so that they can exercise their autonomy in informed decision-making.

Justice is the ethical principle that relates to the distribution of the limited resources of healthcare benefits to the members of society. These resources must be distributed fairly. This issue may arise if there is only one bed left and two delivering mothers. Justice comes into play in deciding which mother should stay and which should be transported or otherwise cared for. The decision should be made according to what is best or most just for the patients and not colored by personal bias.

BENEFICENCE AND NONMALEFICENCE

Beneficence is an ethical principle that involves performing actions that are for the purpose of benefitting another person. In the care of a neonate, any procedure or treatment should be done with the ultimate goal of benefitting the infant, and any actions that are not beneficial should be reconsidered. As the infant ages and/or condition changes, procedures need to be continually reevaluated to determine if they are still of benefit.

Nonmaleficence is an ethical principle that means healthcare workers should provide care in a manner that does not cause direct intentional harm to the patient:

- The actual act must be good or morally neutral.
- The intent must be only for a good effect.
- A bad effect cannot serve as the means to get to a good effect.
- A good effect must have more benefit than a bad effect has harm.

CONFIDENTIALITY

Confidentiality is obligatory in a professional-patient relationship. Nurses are under an obligation to protect the information they possess concerning the patient and family. Care should be taken to safeguard that information and provide the **privacy** that the family deserves. This is accomplished through the use of required passwords when family members call for information about the patient and through the limitation of who is allowed to visit. There may be times when confidentiality must be broken to save the life of a patient, but those circumstances are rare. The nurse must make all efforts to safeguard patient records and identification. Computerized record keeping should be done in such a way that the screen is not visible to others, and paper records must be secured.

> **Review Video: Confidentiality**
> Visit mometrix.com/academy and enter code: 250384

BIOETHICS

Bioethics is a branch of ethics that involves making sure that the medical treatment given is the most **morally correct choice**, given the different options that might be available and the differences inherent in the varied levels of treatment. In the acute/critical care unit, if the patients,

74

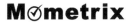

parents, and the staff are in agreement when it comes to values and decision-making, then no ethical dilemma exists; however, when there is a difference in value beliefs between the patients/parents and the staff, there is a **bioethical dilemma** that must be resolved. Sometimes discussion and explanation can resolve differences, but at times, the institution's ethics committee must be brought in to resolve the conflict. The primary goal of bioethics is to determine the most morally correct action using the set of circumstances given.

EMPOWERING FAMILIES TO ACT AS OWN ADVOCATES

Families are empowered to act as their own advocates when they have a clear understanding of their **rights and responsibilities.** These should be given (in print form) and/or presented (audio/video) to parents/guardians on admission or as soon as possible:

- **Rights** should include competent, non-discriminatory medical care that respects privacy and allows participation in decisions about care and the right to refuse care. They should have clear understandable explanations of treatments, options, and conditions, including outcomes. They should be apprised of transfers, changes in care plan, and advance directives. They should have access to medical records information about charges.
- **Responsibilities** should include providing honest and thorough information about health issues and medical history. Parents/guardians should ask for clarification if they don't understand information that is provided to them, and they should follow the plan of care that is outlined or explain why that is not possible. They should treat staff and other patients with respect.

ETHICAL IMPLICATIONS OF GENETIC TESTING IN CHILDREN

Genetic testing poses a number of ethical issues because parents can authorize genetic testing without the consent of the minor. The nurse must serve as an advocate for the infant in cases where genetic testing is done to determine if the child is a carrier or has an adult-onset genetic disease for which there is no cure or adequate treatment, such as Huntington's disease. In both of these cases, the information derived from testing cannot be used for health promotion or disease prevention, so the parents should be counseled to wait until the child is at least in the teen years and can make an informed decision about whether to have testing. This type of information can be devastating to young people who are not provided adequate support and counseling prior to testing. Some people with adult-onset diseases choose not to be tested, and childhood testing robs them of this choice.

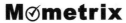

Professional/Legal Issues

INFORMED CONSENT

Parents/guardians of neonates must provide **informed consent** for all treatment the infant receives. This includes a thorough explanation of all procedures and treatment and associated risks. Parents/guardians should be apprised of all options and allowed input on the type of treatments. Parents/guardians should be apprised of all reasonable risks and any complications that might be life threatening or increase morbidity. The American Medical Association has established guidelines for informed consent:

- Explanation of diagnosis.
- Nature and reason for treatment or procedure.
- Risks and benefits.
- Alternative options (regardless of cost or insurance coverage).
- Risks and benefits of alternative options.
- Risks and benefits of not having a treatment or procedure.

Providing informed consent is a requirement of all states.

ADVANCE DIRECTIVES AND DO-NOT-RESUSCITATE ORDERS

In accordance to federal and state laws, individuals have the right to self-determination in health care, including making decisions about end-of-life care through **advance directives,** such as living wills and the right to assign a surrogate person to make decisions through a durable power of attorney. Parents/guardians have the right to make these decisions for minors. Parents/guardians should routinely be questioned about an advanced directive, as they may present at a healthcare organization without the document. If parents/guardians indicate the desire for a **do-not-resuscitate (DNR) order** for a seriously ill child, that child should not receive resuscitative treatments for terminal illness or conditions in which meaningful recovery cannot occur. For those with DNR requests or those withdrawing life support, staff should provide the child palliative rather than curative measures, such as pain control and/or oxygen, and emotional support to the child and family. Religious traditions and beliefs about death should be treated with respect.

NEGLIGENCE

Risk management must attempt to determine the burden of proof for acts of **negligence**, including compliance with duty, breaches in procedures, degree of harm, and cause. Negligence indicates that *proper care* has not been provided, based on established standards. *Reasonable care* uses rationales for decision-making in relation to providing care. State regulations regarding negligence may vary, but all have some statutes of limitations. There are a number of different types of negligence:

- **Negligent conduct**, meaning that an individual failed to provide reasonable care or to protect/assist another, based on standards and expertise.
- **Gross negligence**, or willfully providing inadequate care while disregarding the safety and security of another.
- **Contributory negligence**, in which the injured party has contributed to his/her own harm.
- **Comparative negligence**, which attributing a percentage of negligence to each individual involved.

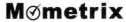

EMR

The **electronic medical record** (EMR) is a digital computerized patient record, which may be integrated with CPOE and CDSS to improve patient care and reduce medical error. Software applications vary considerably, and standardization has not yet been implemented, so the organization must carefully review current and future anticipated needs, as well as the ability of applications to interface with each other to provide for adequate measurements, data collection, reports, data retrieval, analysis, and confidentiality. Increasingly, physicians in private practice, especially those in large groups, are employing EMRs, which may be different systems from those used in hospitals. Systems can be customized to meet the needs of the organization, but cost and lack of standardization remain barriers to implementation. However, studies indicate that there is a positive correlation between comprehensive EMR systems and patient outcomes. Quantifiable data about cost-effectiveness can be difficult to calculate because savings are often in terms of saved time, fewer interventions, and reduced error.

DOCUMENTATION

Documentation is a form of communication that provides information about the healthcare patient and confirms that care was provided. Accurate, objective, and complete documentation of patient care is required by both accreditation and reimbursement agencies, including federal and state governments. Purposes of documentation include:

- Carrying out professional responsibility.
- Establishing accountability.
- Communicating among health professionals.
- Educating staff.
- Providing information for research.
- Satisfying legal and practice standards.
- Ensuring reimbursement.

While documentation focuses on progress notes, there are many other aspects to charting. Doctors' orders must be noted, medication administration must be documented on medication sheets, and vital signs must be graphed. Flow sheets must be checked off, filled out, or initialed. Admission assessments may involve primarily checklists or may require extensive documentation. The primary issue in malpractice cases is inaccurate or incomplete documentation. It's better to over-document than under-document, but effective documentation does neither.

PROFESSIONAL ORGANIZATIONS

Many **professional pediatric nursing organizations** are available for neonatal nurses to join. A professional organization is a group of practitioners who share a common interest. They are able to form a collective voice that can influence standards of practice, institutional policies, and governing regulations and laws. They may have admission standards for those wishing to join and provide ethical guidelines for members. Other benefits often include educational opportunities in a chosen area of specialty, newsletters concerning healthcare trends and issues that affect their specialty area, and gatherings where peers meet for discussions. Some organizations available for neonatal nurses include:

- The Academy of Neonatal Nurses (ANN).
- The Association of Women's Health, Obstetric, and Neonatal Nurses (AWHONN).
- The National Association of Neonatal Nurses (NANN).
- The National Association of Pediatric Nurse Practitioners (NAPNP).

HIPAA

The **Health Insurance Portability and Accountability Act** (HIPAA) addresses the rights of the individual related to the **privacy of health information**. A nurse must not release any information or documentation about a patient's condition or treatment without **consent**, as the individual has the right to determine who has access to personal information. Personal information about the patient is considered **protected health information (PHI)** and consists of any identifying or personal information about the patient, such as health history, condition, or treatments in any form, and any documentation, including electronic, verbal, or written. Personal information can be shared with spouse, legal guardians, those with durable power of attorney for the patient, and those involved in care of the patient, such as physicians, without a specific release, but the patient should always be consulted if personal information is to be discussed with others present to ensure that there is no objection. Failure to comply with HIPAA regulations can make a nurse liable for legal action.

EMTALA

The **Emergency Medical Treatment and Active Labor Act** (EMTALA) is designed to prevent patient "dumping" from emergency departments (ED) and is an issue of concern for risk management, requiring staff training for compliance:

- Transfers from the ED may be intra-hospital or to another facility.
- Stabilization of the patient with emergency conditions or active labor must be done in the ED prior to transfer, and initial screening must be given prior to inquiring about insurance or ability to pay.
- Stabilization requires treatment for emergency conditions and reasonable belief that, although the emergency condition may not be completely resolved, the patient's condition will not deteriorate during transfer.
- Women in the ED in active labor should deliver both the child and placenta before transfer.
- The receiving department or facility should be capable of treating the patient and dealing with complications that might occur.
- Transfer to another facility is indicated if the patient requires specialized services not available within the hospital, such as to burn centers.

Nurse Practice Act

Each state has its own **nurse practice act,** which is administered through regulations by the state Board of Nursing. The nurse practice act outlines requirements for licensure and certification and delineates the scope of practice of nurses, including duties and delegation. Typically, licensure is granted to those who complete an accredited LVN/LPN or RN program and pass the nursing exam (NCLEX) or receive endorsement because of licensure in another state. RN programs may be 3-year hospital-based programs, associate degree or bachelor's degree. Foreign-trained nurses may need to meet special requirements that are determined by the state Board of Nursing and included in the nurse practice act. The nurse practice act of each state provides the requirement for advanced practice certification and the professional designation. Additionally, the nurse practice acts outline the requirements for relicensing or recertification, often including the need for continuing education. The nurse practice act also includes provisions for disciplinary action.

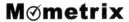

NURSE-PATIENT RATIOS

Nurse-patient ratios refer to the number of patients assigned to a nurse. For example, if one nurse is assigned responsibility for 4 patients, the ratio is 1:4. Ratios are an area of concern because studies have consistently shown better outcomes for patients with lower nurse-patient ratios. However, the lower the ratio, the higher the costs. Only California currently has mandated nurse-patient ratios. The California law, often cited as a model, requires a 1:1 ratio in the operating room and for trauma patients in the ER, 1:2 in ICU, NICU, post-anesthesia recovery, labor and delivery, and ICU patients in the ER. Ratios in other areas range from 1:3 to 1:6 (the maximum). Massachusetts has a mandate for ICU only, 1:1 or 1:2. A number of other states require staffing committees to establish staffing policies, and some states require public reporting of nurse-patient ratios even though they do not mandate the ratios.

Patient Safety

IMPORTANCE OF COMMUNICATION IN PATIENT SAFETY

Many adverse incidents related to **patient safety** result from errors or failures in **communication**. In fact, over 30% of malpractice claims result from communication failures. Communication is especially a concern during hand-off procedures. Critical information about the patient may be undocumented, forgotten, overlooked, or misplaced. For this reason, standardized hand-off procedures, such as SBAR (**S**ituation, **B**ackground, **A**ssessment, **R**ecommendation) or I-PASS (**I**llness severity, **P**atient summary, **A**ction list, **S**ituation awareness/contingency planning, **S**ynthesis by receiver) should be utilized. While an initial error in communication may not directly harm a patient, the decisions made by subsequent healthcare providers may cause harm because the healthcare providers lacked essential information. Additionally, communication failures may occur because healthcare providers don't take the time to talk with patients or family or to listen attentively and to gather their input. Problems may arise if healthcare providers fail to document medications, treatments, or observations in a timely manner. Many electronic health records utilize limited narration in favor of checklists, and checking all the boxes may become a rote activity, leading to errors.

COUNSELING TECHNIQUES FOR FAMILIES WITH NEONATES IN NICU

Counseling techniques for families and extended families with a neonate in the NICU include:

- **Talk with families and listen:** Assess the family members' understanding of the neonate's condition and the situation and determine if it is realistic or distorted. If distorted, try to ascertain the reason and provide useful information in a non-threatening manner to help them to more fully understand but avoid overwhelming family members with too much information, especially initially. Listen attentively and show respect at all times. Acknowledge family members feeling of guilt and explain these feelings are normal. Pay attention to body language when delivering information.
- **Assess coping strategies/grief:** Determine how the family members cope with stress and handle grief and provide support and information about resources and support groups that are available and may be appropriate.
- **Encourage expression of feelings:** Remain supportive of family members' feelings and responses, even if negative, and encourage them to interact and share feelings with others. Suggest keeping a journal, diary, or blog to write about their feelings and experiences.

SHARED DECISION-MAKING AND PARENT-STAFF DISAGREEMENTS

Issues that arise in the NICU include:

- **Shared decision making:** Requires that staff members treat the parents with respect, listen to their opinions and feelings, provide full information about treatments and the neonate's condition, encourage the parents to participate in care, and encourage parents to collaborate and share in decision-making at every step in the NICU provision of care.
- **Parent-staff disagreements:** When disagreements occur between parents and staff members, it's important to respond with patience and empathy. The nurse should try to determine why the parents disagree or are angry. For example, are they afraid a treatment is harmful, do they not understand, have they been reading advice on the internet or getting advice from others, have they developed a dislike or distrust for staff members, do they feel left out of decision making, do they resent lack of control, or is a treatment at odds with their cultural beliefs? The staff members should ask parents what they want and why and provide as complete information as possible, including pros and cons.

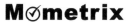

INTERPROFESSIONAL PRACTICE

Interprofessional practice often begins with interprofessional education in which members of two or more professions study and learn together in order to build relationships and to have a better understanding of the contributions of each profession and the role of the profession in ensuring patient safety. For example, in neonatal nursing, an interprofessional group may include a physician, nurse, midwife, ultrasonographer, respiratory therapist, radiologist, pharmacist, nutritionist, and breastfeeding specialist. Each has a different but equally important role in patient care. A better understanding of roles and responsibilities leads to better collaboration and fewer patient safety issues. Additionally, collaboration promotes cross training and awareness of patient needs. Key elements in interprofessional practice include leadership (definitions, who leads and how leadership is determined), monitoring (continually assessing processes and outcomes), communication (methods and styles of effective communication), and support (mutual and organizational). Studies indicate that interprofessional education and practice especially improves communication among participants, a critical element in patient safety.

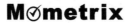

Quality Improvement

EVIDENCE-BASED RESEARCH

Evidence-based research is the use of current research and patient values in practice to establish a plan of care for each patient. Research may be the result of large studies of best practices or individual research from observations in practice about the effectiveness of treatment. Evidence-based practice requires a commitment to ongoing research and outcomes evaluations. Evidence-based practice requires a thorough understanding of research methods in order to evaluate the results and determine if they can be generalized. Results must also be evaluated in terms of cost-effectiveness. Steps to evidence-based practice include:

- Making a diagnosing.
- Researching and analyzing results.
- Applying research findings to plan of care.
- Evaluating outcomes.

Incorporating research findings should be central to all work of the nurse and should be routinely disseminated as part of practice, education, and consultation. Research findings should be used as the basis for evidence-based practice.

CRITICAL READING/EVALUATION OF RESEARCH

There are a number of steps to **critical reading/evaluation** of research:

- **Consider the source** of the material. If it is in the popular press, it may have little validity compared to something published in a juried journal.
- **Review the author's credentials** to determine if a person is an expert in the field of study.
- **Determine thesis,** or the central claim of the research. It should be clearly stated.
- **Examine the organization** of the article, whether it is based on a particular theory, and the type of methodology used.
- **Review the evidence** to determine how it is used to support the main points. Look for statistical evidence and sample size to determine if the findings have wide applicability.
- **Evaluate** the overall article to determine if the information seems credible and useful and should be communicated to administration and/or staff.

SELECTION AND INFORMATION BIAS

Selection bias occurs when the method of selecting subjects results in a cohort that is not representative of the target population because of inherent error in design. For example, if all infants who develop urinary infections are evaluated per urine culture and sensitivities for microbial resistance, but only those infants with clinically-evident infections are included, a number of patients with sub-clinical infections may be missed, skewing the results. Selection bias is only a concern when participants in studies are specifically chosen. Many surveillance studies do not involve selection of subjects.

Information bias occurs when there are errors in classification, so an estimate of association is incorrect. Non-differential misclassification occurs when there is similar misclassification of disease or exposure among both those who are diseased/exposed and those who are not. Differential misclassification occurs when there is a differing misclassification of disease or exposure among both those who are diseased/exposed and those who are not.

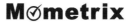

INTERNAL AND EXTERNAL VALIDITY

Many research studies are most concerned with **internal validity**, adequate unbiased data properly collected and analyzed within the population studied, but studies that determine the efficacy of procedures or treatments, for example, should have **external validity** as well; that is, the results should be **generalizable** (true) for similar populations. **Replication** of the study with different subjects, researchers, and under different circumstances should produce similar results. For various reasons, some people may be excluded from a study so that instead of randomized subjects, the subjects may be highly selected so when data is compared with another population in which there is less or more selection, results may be different. The selection of subjects, in this case, would interfere with external validity. Part of the design of a study should include considerations of whether or not it should have external validity or whether there is value for the institution based solely on internal validation.

HYPOTHESIS AND HYPOTHESIS TESTING

A **hypothesis** should be generated about the probable cause of the disease/infection based on the information available in laboratory and medical records, epidemiologic study, literature review, and expert opinion. A hypothesis, for example, should include the infective agent, the likely source, and the mode of transmission: "Wound infections with *Staphylococcus aureus* were caused by reuse and inadequate sterilization of single-use irrigation syringes used during wound care in the NICU."

Hypothesis testing includes data analysis, laboratory findings, and outcomes of environmental testing. It usually includes **case control studies**, with 2-4 controls picked for each case of infection. They may be matched according to age, sex, or other characteristics, but they are not infected at the time they are picked for the study. **Cohort studies**, whose controls are picked based on having or lacking exposure, may also be instituted. If the hypothesis cannot be supported, then a new hypothesis or different testing methods may be necessary.

OUTCOMES EVALUATION

Outcomes evaluation is an important component of evidence-based practice, which involves both internal and external research. All treatments are subjected to review to determine if they produce positive outcomes, and policies and protocols for outcomes evaluation should be in place. Outcomes evaluation includes the following:

- **Monitoring** over the course of treatment involves careful observation and record keeping that notes progress, with supporting laboratory and radiographic evidence as indicated by condition and treatment.
- **Evaluating** results includes reviewing records as well as current research to determine if outcomes are within acceptable parameters.
- **Sustaining** involves continuing treatment, but continuing to monitor and evaluate.
- **Improving** means to continue the treatment but with additions or modifications in order to improve outcomes.
- **Replacing** the treatment with a different treatment must be done if outcomes evaluation indicates that current treatment is ineffective.

Low Risk Neonatal Practice Test

1. A neonate is at risk of developing congenital varicella syndrome if the mother became infected

    a. in the first 20 weeks of pregnancy

    b. after the first 20 weeks of pregnancy

    c. during the last week of pregnancy

2. Asymmetric intrauterine growth restriction is caused by problems that occur during the

    a. first trimester

    b. second trimester

    c. third trimester

3. A preterm neonate has persistent episodes of apnea lasting greater than 20 seconds resulting in heart rate of 76 bpm and pallor/cyanosis, suggesting apnea of prematurity. The drug of choice to stimulate respirations is

    a. indomethacin

    b. caffeine

    c. doxapram

4. A nevus flammeus (port-wine stain) birthmark is characterized by

    a. blue-black discoloration on the buttocks and dorsal area

    b. raised demarcated dark red lesion

    c. unraised demarcated red-purple lesion

5. Before a heelstick to obtain a blood sample, the most appropriate method of pain control that can be utilized is

    a. oral acetaminophen

    b. a sucrose-dipped pacifier

    c. topical anesthetic

6. An indication for vacuum-assisted delivery of a fetus is

    a. extended second stage of labor

    b. advanced cranial molding

    c. uncertain fetal station

7. An important advantage of interprofessional practice is

    a. clearer definition of roles

    b. decreased workload

    c. improved communication

8. A mother's smoking during pregnancy places the fetus at increased risk of

    a. low birth weight

    b. renal abnormalities

    c. bradycardia

9. If a pregnant woman has chlamydia, vaginal delivery of the neonate may result in

    a. skin infection

    b. eye and lung infections

    c. genitourinary infection

10. An umbilical vein catheter is more appropriate than an arterial vein catheter for infusions of

    a. drugs

    b. fluids

    c. packed red blood cells

11. If a mother suffers from pregnancy-induced hypertension (preeclampsia) during pregnancy, the primary detrimental effect on the fetus is

    a. intrauterine growth restriction (IUGR)

    b. placental abruption

    c. spontaneous abortion

12. When conducting a review of the literature as part of evidence-based research, the level of evidence that is based on a quasi-experimental study, such as a matched case-control study, would be categorized as

    a. level I

    b. level II

    c. level III

13. If a neonate is exposed to repeated alarms and is exhibiting less reaction to the sound, this is an indication of

    a. self-regulating

    b. habituation

    c. attentional response

14. A neonate born to an HIV-infected mother should receive the first dose of antiretroviral medication within

    a. 6 to 12 hours after birth

    b. 6 to 12 weeks after birth

    c. 1 year after birth

15. If a patient has gestational diabetes that is well-controlled and without complications, induction is often carried out at

    a. 36 weeks

    b. 38 weeks

    c. 40 weeks

16. When a neonate is diagnosed with a terminal disease, the mother cries inconsolably, but the father appears detached and calm. The father's reaction is probably an indication of

    a. anticipatory grief

    b. delayed grief

    c. incongruent grief

17. To promote family integration, the best time for siblings to visit the mother and neonate is

    a. as soon after delivery as possible

    b. just prior to discharge from hospital

    c. after discharge from hospital

18. Critical congenital heart disease screening (CCHD) is carried out on the newborn through physical examination and

    a. ECG

    b. ultrasound

    c. pulse oximetry

19. In the nonstress test (NST), fetal heart rate acceleration without movement probably indicates

    a. adequate oxygenation

    b. fetal hypoxemia

    c. fetal metabolic acidosis

20. A neonate is exhibiting airway compromise. The bronchodilator that is likely to have the fewest adverse effects is

    a. albuterol

    b. theophylline

    c. levalbuterol

21. If a quad screen shows high AFT, and normal hCG, uE^3 and INH-A, this indicates

    a. neural tube defect

    b. trisomy 21

    c. multiple gestation

22. If a Haitian woman states she does not want to name her baby girl, the nurse should assume

    a. the woman is not bonding with the neonate

    b. delayed naming is a cultural norm

    c. the woman is unhappy with the child's gender

23. When placing a newborn in a safety car seat, the seat should be rear-facing and

    a. reclined 30-45 degrees

    b. upright

    c. flat

24. The type of neonatal drug testing that universally detects the most drugs and for the longest duration of time is

    a. urine

    b. hair

    c. meconium

25. With electronic fetal monitoring, an abrupt variable deceleration often indicates

    a. cord compression
    b. fetal demise
    c. maternal hypotension

26. The neonatal hearing test that measures the integrity of the middle and inner ear and the outer hair cells of the cochlea is the

    a. auditory brainstem response
    b. otoacoustic emissions test
    c. bone-conduction test

27. In a frank breech position, the fetal legs

    a. precede the buttocks into the maternal pelvis
    b. are in flexed position against the abdomen and chest
    c. extend across the abdomen toward the shoulders

28. By two hours after birth, the neonate's PaO_2 should have stabilized at

    a. 80 to 95 mm Hg
    b. 33 to 85 mm Hg
    c. 8 to 24 mm Hg

29. An early indication of maternal hemorrhage is often

    a. decreased blood pressure
    b. maternal bradycardia
    c. fetal bradycardia or tachycardia

30. A pregnant patient with BP 150/100, proteinuria 0.5 g in a 24-hour specimen, normal platelet count, and normal urinary output with no complaints of pain would be classified as having

    a. hypertension
    b. mild preeclampsia
    c. severe preeclampsia

31. Consistent late decelerations are almost always an indication of

    a. epidural anesthetic
    b. preeclampsia
    c. uteroplacental insufficiency

32. During induction of labor with oxytocin, if hypertonic contractions develop, the initial response should be to

    a. reduce or discontinue oxytocin
    b. reposition the patient
    c. administer oxygen at 8 to 10 L/min

33. The three levels of motor organization are

    a. muscles, nerves, and brain
    b. spinal cord, brain stem, and cerebral cortex
    c. spinal cord, nerves, cerebral cortex

34. The HELLP syndrome is characterized by (H) hemolysis, (EL) elevated liver enzymes, and (LP)

   a. lateral pain

   b. low (blood) pressure

   c. low platelet count

35. Conditions associated with oligohydramnios include

   a. urinary tract anomalies

   b. chromosomal abnormalities, such as trisomy 21

   c. obstructional lesions of GI tract

36. A new mother notes that her neonate often seems restless and sleeps about 12 out of 24 hours. This amount of sleep is

   a. normal

   b. inadequate

   c. excessive

37. If the biophysical profile shows a score of 8 with normal amniotic fluid volume, the required intervention is

   a. no intervention needed

   b. induction of labor

   c. repeat test the same day

38. A neonate who was exposed to maternal opioid drugs prenatally is undergoing neonatal abstinence syndrome with NAS scores of 9 three times consecutively (Finnegan scale), indicating the need for medical treatment. The drug of choice is generally

   a. clonidine

   b. phenobarbital

   c. tincture of opium (diluted)

39. Within 2 to 3 hours of birth, a newborn's temperature should stabilize at

   a. 36.5-37 °C (97.7-98.6 °F)

   b. 35.5-36.4 °C (96-97.5 °F)

   c. 34.5-35.4 °C (94-95.7 °F)

40. If a newborn with myelomeningocele has passed no urine in more than 24 hours, the most likely reason is

   a. neurogenic bladder

   b. urethral obstruction

   c. dehydration

41. A new mother should be advised that, by day 4 after birth, a neonate should urinate approximately

   a. 3 times daily

   b. 6 times daily

   c. 10 times daily

42. The most common complication of multiple births is

    a. birth defects
    b. twin-to-twin transfusion syndrome
    c. preterm birth

43. In a neonate, pathological jaundice is usually evident

    a. at birth
    b. within the first 24 hours after birth
    c. within the first 24 to 48 hours after birth

44. On day one of birth for a term infant, the normal blood glucose level should be

    a. 40 to 60 mg/dL (2.2 to 3.3 mmol/L)
    b. 50 to 80 mg/dL (2.8 to 4.4 mmol/L)
    c. 60 to 100 mg/dL (3.3 to 5.6 mmol/L)

45. According to Safe Sleep guidelines, parents should be taught to place a neonate on the back

    a. when the neonate is sleeping and unattended
    b. during the night
    c. during the first two weeks

46. The correct position of the neonate for Kangaroo Care is the neonate

    a. lying tightly swathed in mother's arm in breastfeeding position
    b. lying upright between mother's bare breasts
    c. being carried in a sling about the mother's waist

47. Ensuring that a woman has given informed consent and understands her rights and all of the risks and benefits of a procedure or treatment supports the ethical principal of

    a. beneficence
    b. nonmaleficence
    c. autonomy

48. On the New Ballard Score for assessment of gestational age, a score of zero (0) indicates

    a. 20 weeks gestation
    b. 24 weeks gestation
    c. 40 weeks gestation

49. The most common reason for elevated bilirubin levels within a week of birth in a breastfed infant is

    a. fatty acids resulting from cold stress
    b. inadequate intake of human milk
    c. immature gastrointestinal tract

50. Fetal bradycardia with variable decelerations during uterine contractions may indicate

    a. placenta previa
    b. abruptio placentae
    c. prolapsed cord

51. A neonate has had frequent blood draws to monitor electrolyte and glucose levels. Phlebotomy has caused anemia of prematurity (AOP) although the infant is not acutely hypoxemic. The initial treatment is

    a. recombinant human erythropoietin (rHuEPO)
    b. fresh frozen platelets (FFP)
    c. platelets

52. Placing the newborn infant against the mother's bare skin helps to reduce

    a. evaporative heat loss
    b. conductive heat loss
    c. convective heat loss

53. A neonate has been diagnosed with craniotabes because of a softened area of skull in the posterior occipital area. The most likely treatment is

    a. observation
    b. AV shunt
    c. protective helmet

54. With acute respiratory distress syndrome (ARDS) in the neonate, the goal of therapy is to maintain oxygen saturation at

    a. >85%
    b. >90%
    c. >95%

55. Early-onset sepsis (≤72 hours) in the neonate most often presents as

    a. bacteremia
    b. meningitis
    c. pneumonia

56. When treating a neonate for hypothermia, the air temperature should be increased by approximately

    a. 0.5 °C every hour until infant stabilizes
    b. 1 °C every hour until infant stabilizes
    c. 2 °C every hour until infant stabilizes

57. A full term neonate fails to pass meconium in the first 48 hours of life. The infant exhibits abdominal distension, poor feeding, and bilious vomiting. An x-ray of the abdomen shows dilated loops of bowel. The diagnostic procedure used both to confirm a diagnosis of meconium plug syndrome and to treat is

    a. MRI
    b. colonoscopy
    c. contrast enema

58. Edema of the fetal scalp resulting from pressure of the head against the cervix is

    a. cephalohematoma
    b. caput succedaneum
    c. molding

59. During the initial physical examination, the neonate's chest circumference is 34 cm. The expected head circumference is

    a. 32 cm
    b. 34 cm
    c. 36 cm

60. A neonate is 40 weeks of gestation and nursing well but has onset of jaundice at 36 hours. Total serum bilirubin is 12 mg/dL. At this time, treatment should include

    a. continued observation and jaundice assessment
    b. phototherapy
    c. exchange transfusion

61. A neonate at 37 weeks of gestation is born to a mother who has abused cocaine throughout pregnancy. The neonate exhibits persistent hypertonia, startles easily, and shows signs of distress at any disturbance. The most appropriate treatment is

    a. anticonvulsant
    b. sedative
    c. swaddling and reduction in external stimuli

62. When evaluating cord blood values 30 minutes after birth, the arterial PO_2 that is within normal limits is

    a. 28-32 mmHg
    b. 16-20 mmHg
    c. 40-50 mmHg

63. A neonate, 2 days after birth, develops a generalized rash with erythematous papules, vesicles, and some pustules everywhere but on the palms and soles of feet. The most likely diagnosis is

    a. erythema toxicum
    b. neonatal pustular melanosis
    c. cutis marmorata

64. A mother delivers a child with sickle cell disease, an autosomal recessive disorder. The recurrence risk for subsequent children being born with the disorder is

    a. 25% for each pregnancy and 50% chance the child will become a carrier
    b. 50% for each pregnancy and 25% chance the child will become a carrier
    c. 50% for each pregnancy and no carrier state

65. A neonate born with the genetic disorder cystic fibrosis must be monitored carefully for

    a. apnea
    b. hypoglycemia
    c. meconium ileus

66. A neonate develops tremors of the chin and extremities with the following:

- Lack of ocular deviations or other abnormalities.
- Gentle restraint halts tremors.
- Stimulation elicits tremors.
- Clonic jerking has both fast and slow elements.
- Autonomic changes involving the heart rate, respirations, and blood pressure are not present.
- EEG is normal.

The most likely cause is
   a. jitteriness
   b. seizures
   c. shivering

67. A neonate exhibits signs of hypoglycemia after birth and is treated only with a bolus of glucose. This treatment puts the infant at risk for
   a. bolus-associated hyperglycemia
   b. bolus-associated hypoglycemia
   c. hyperinsulinism

68. On examining the neonate, the neonatal nurse practitioner notes 9 café au lait spots with a diameter greater than 5 mm and freckles on the axilla and inguinal area. The infant should be tested for
   a. neurofibromatosis, type 1
   b. Sturge-Weber syndrome
   c. Addison's disease

69. A neonate who was exposed to maternal herpes virus should be treated to with
   a. nothing, as no treatment is effective
   b. IV acyclovir
   c. topical acyclovir

70. The type of hearing loss associated with *in utero* rubella infection is
   a. conductive
   b. central
   c. sensorineural

71. Asymmetry in gluteal and thigh creases in a neonate may indicate
   a. hip dysplasia
   b. spina bifida occulta
   c. cerebellar ataxia

72. On auscultating the neonate's heart sounds, the S1 sound is louder than normal. This may be an indication of
   a. congestive heart failure
   b. ventricular septal defect
   c. aortic stenosis

73. When assessing the plantar grasp reflex in a neonate, a normal response is

    a. toes remain in neutral position

    b. extension of the toes

    c. flexion of the toes

74. Meconium was detected in the amniotic fluid during delivery of a neonate. At birth, the infant is hypotonic and respiration are depressed. The infant should be placed on a radiant warmer and

    a. endotracheal suctioning performed

    b. mouth cleared of secretions with bulb syringe

    c. positive pressure ventilation performed

75. All HIV-exposed neonates whose mothers took antiretroviral drugs during pregnancy should receive HIV prophylaxis after delivery with

    a. both zidovudine and nevirapine

    b. nevirapine

    c. zidovudine

76. Inhaled nitrous oxide (iNO) may be used as an inhaled pulmonary vasodilator for neonates with

    a. persistent pulmonary hypertension of the newborn

    b. pulmonic stenosis

    c. chronic lung disease

77. Following birth, damage to the neonate's upper brachial plexus (C5 to C7) is likely to result in

    a. ipsilateral Horner syndrome

    b. Klumpke's palsy

    c. Erb's palsy

78. A neonate that suffered birth trauma with hypoxemia developed firm reddened circumscribed nodules in fatty areas of the body about 7 days after birth and is diagnosed with fat necrosis. The electrolyte that should be monitored closely is

    a. sodium

    b. calcium

    c. potassium

79. If a neonate's cardiac status appeared normal at birth but 48 hours later the neonate experiences a precipitous drop in circulation to the lower body, the likely congenital heart defect is

    a. ventricular septal defect

    b. aortic stenosis

    c. coarctation of the aorta

80. Necrotizing enterocolitis in a preterm infant is usually caused by

    a. ischemic bowel

    b. severe constipation

    c. generalized infection

81. **If a neonate has a patent ductus arteriosus, the usual initial treatment is**
    a. captopril
    b. prostaglandin
    c. indomethacin

82. **Most neonates pass the first meconium within**
    a. 6 hours of birth
    b. 24 hours of birth
    c. 48 hours of birth

83. **If bloody mucoid discharge is noted in a newborn's vaginal area, this is a(n)**
    a. normal finding
    b. sign of congenital abnormality
    c. indication of infection

84. **Preterm infants are at risk of hyperkalemia primarily because of**
    a. inadequate intake
    b. potassium shift
    c. excessive supplementation

85. **On examination, a newborn is found to have a scrotal mass that is soft and painless and does not change in size but transilluminates, probably indicating a(n)**
    a. inguinal hernia
    b. scrotal tumor
    c. hydrocele

86. **Small urate crystals found in the urine of a newborn are a sign of**
    a. immature renal function
    b. renal failure
    c. urinary infection

87. **Newborns tend to regurgitate after feeding because the**
    a. stomach contracts forcefully
    b. emptying of gastric contents is delayed
    c. gastroesophageal sphincter is immature

88. **If a newborn has metatarsus adductus ("toeing in") of 20 degrees in both feet, the likely treatment is**
    a. foot braces
    b. surgical repair
    c. serial long-leg casting

89. **If a 7-day-old newborn begins crying frantically and exhibits scrotal swelling and negative cremasteric reflex, the most likely cause is**
    a. inguinal hernia
    b. testicular torsion
    c. hydrocele

90. Transient tachypnea of the newborn (TTN) occurs because of

a. aspiration of amniotic fluid
b. CNS depression
c. fluid in the lungs not adequately absorbed

91. An increased risk factor for pneumothorax in the newborn is caused by

a. meconium aspiration
b. maternal eclampsia
c. post-term birth

92. The type of seizures that are the most common in newborns is

a. subtle
b. clonic
c. tonic

93. Two weeks after birth, a newborn develops bulging fontanels, bradycardia, hypotension and abnormal dolls-eye reflex, suggesting

a. subarachnoid hemorrhage
b. subdural hemorrhage
c. epidural hemorrhage

94. The purpose of a partial exchange transfusion for a newborn with polycythemia is to lower the hematocrit to

a. 55 to 60%
b. 50 to 55%
c. 45 to 50%

95. If a breastfeeding mother develops painful cracked nipples, the most likely cause is

a. breastfeeding for extended periods
b. infection
c. improper latching on

96. If an intraventricular hemorrhage (IVH) extends 50% or more into the lateral ventricles of the brain with significant dilation of the ventricles, the IVH is classified as

a. grade II
b. grade III
c. grade IV

97. A newborn's hemoglobin from cord blood should be approximately

a. 16.8 g/dL (168 mmol/L)
b. 19.8 g/dL (198 mmol/L)
c. 20 g/dL (200 mmol/L)

98. A neonate has abdominal distention, bilious vomiting, diarrhea with bloody stools, tachycardia, tachypnea, and cycles of cramping pain every 15 to 30 minutes. These symptoms are consistent with

a. Hirschsprung disease
b. intussusception
c. volvulus

99. A scrotal mass that may be reduced with gentle pressure is likely a(n)

    a. inguinal hernia
    b. scrotal tumor
    c. hydrocele

100. A finding that may indicate an alcohol-related birth defect is

    a. flattened occiput
    b. micrognathia
    c. broad nasal bridge

101. A mother had previous breast reduction surgery and wants to breastfeed her neonate but her milk supply remains at about 75% of normal production. The most effective solution is to

    a. switch to formula feedings
    b. alternate breastfeeding and bottle feeding
    c. utilize a nursing supplementation system

102. If natal teeth are noted on the newborn's physical examination,

    a. further evaluation is necessary
    b. this is a normal benign finding
    c. the teeth must be extracted

103. If a woman was infected with Zika virus at some point during pregnancy, the fetus is at risk for

    a. hydrocephalus
    b. microcephaly
    c. anencephaly

104. A neonate has developed gastroesophageal reflux disease, regurgitating frequently after eating. The mother has been told to hold the infants at a 45-60° angle for breastfeeding. After feeding, the infant should be

    a. placed in prone position
    b. held upright in the arms for 30 minutes
    c. placed upright in an infant seat for 30 minutes

105. The type of heat loss that occurs when a newborn is placed on a cold scale is

    a. evaporative
    b. convective
    c. conductive

106. An infant is classified as large for gestational age (LGA) if the weight is

    a. above the 90th percentile
    b. above the 85th percentile
    c. above the 75th percentile

107. During assessment of the Moro ("startle") reflex, a normal response is for the newborn to

    a. extend the arms and flex the legs
    b. flex the arms and extend the legs
    c. extend the arms and the legs

108. If a newborn has been breastfeeding readily and urinating but has abdominal distention and no passage of stool in 36 hours after birth, the newborn should be assessed for

    a. constipation
    b. imperforate anus
    c. intestinal infection

109. If a neonate is born with gastroschisis, the exposed organs should be

    a. pushed back into place and covered with dry dressing
    b. irrigated and covered with wet dressings
    c. covered with moist gauze and wrapped in plastic

110. A neonate has the characteristic physical differences associated with trisomy 21 (Down syndrome). The neonate should be further evaluated for

    a. congenital heart disease
    b. pyloric stenosis
    c. ambiguous genitalia

111. If a newborn that has been circumcised urinates, the area should be cleansed with

    a. soap and water
    b. baby wipes
    c. water only.

112. If the newborn's color is good when the mouth is open but becomes cyanotic when the mouth is closed, this may indicate

    a. choanal atresia
    b. deviated septum
    c. respiratory distress syndrome

113. In order to prevent transmission of Group B *Streptococcus* to a neonate, an infected mother in labor needs at least

    a. one dose of antibiotic
    b. 4 hours of antibiotic therapy
    c. 8 hours of antibiotic therapy

114. The most likely treatment for a newborn that suffered a right clavicular fracture during a breech birth is

    a. immobilization of the arm
    b. surgical repair
    c. no treatment necessary

115. A newborn is classified as small for gestational age (SGA) if the weight is

    a. less than the 25th percentile

    b. less than the 20th percentile

    c. less than the 10th percentile

116. When placing a temperature probe on a supine neonate to monitor thermoregulation, a good location for the probe is over the

    a. mid-scapular region of the back

    b. liver

    c. mediastinum

117. The relationship between the total loading dose of an administered drug and the serum concentration refers to the

    a. absorption

    b. distribution

    c. clearance

118. The percentage of calories from carbohydrates in human milk is

    a. 40%

    b. 60%

    c. 80%

119. A normal finding when assessing a neonate's fontanels is

    a. fontanels are slightly below level of skull

    b. fontanels bulge slightly above level of skull

    c. fontanels are level with skull

120. Respiratory acidosis is characterized by

    a. hyperventilation and increased excretion of CO_2

    b. hypoventilation and CO_2 retention

    c. decreased serum pH and PCO_2

121. The method of feeding that poses the fewest problems for a newborn with cleft lip and palate is

    a. breastfeeding

    b. bottle feeding

    c. enteral feeding

122. A contraindication to breastfeeding is

    a. maternal HIV positive status

    b. maternal infection with hepatitis C

    c. active maternal smoking

123. Compensated metabolic acidosis is characterized by

    a. increase serum pH and decreased PCO_2

    b. increased serum pH and PCO_2

    c. decreased serum pH and PCO_2

124. During lactation, a woman usually requires an additional

   a. 200 calories per day
   b. 500 calories per day
   c. 1000 calories per day

125. Erythromycin ointment should be administered into the newborn's eyes after birth at least within

   a. 10 minutes
   b. 1 hour
   c. 12 hours

126. If a woman who is breastfeeding asks when to start providing supplementary feedings, the woman should be advised to wait for at least

   a. 2 months
   b. 4 months
   c. 6 months

127. During resuscitation of a distressed hypoxic, bradycardic neonate, the compression-ventilation ratio should be

   a. 3:1
   b. 4:1
   c. 5:1

128. The type of human milk that provides passive immunity to the neonate is

   a. colostrum
   b. transitional
   c. mature foremilk

129. After a neonate is resuscitated using a bag and mask and stabilized, the infant then requires

   a. positive pressure ventilation
   b. gastric suctioning
   c. oxygen administration via nasal cannula

130. At three days postpartum, the mother has developed painfully engorged breasts. To relieve the engorgement, the mother should

   a. use a breast pump to reduce engorgement
   b. apply warm compresses
   c. increase nursing frequency to every 2 to 3 hours

131. When treating a neonate with hyperbilirubinemia with phototherapy, the lights should be above the neonate at a distance of

   a. 10 to 15 cm
   b. 15 to 20 cm
   c. 25 to 35 cm

132. A mother brings her term infant (and first child) for an exam at 2 weeks after birth. The baby has not regained birth weight, appears listless, face drawn, and skin turgor is poor. The mother is breastfeeding. The most appropriate first action is

   a. questioning mother about nursing technique and frequency and observing the infant nursing
   b. reporting the mother to child protective services for neglect
   c. advising the mother to stop breastfeeding and switch to formula

133. A female neonate is born with cystic hygroma (webbing) of the neck, swelling of distal extremities, low-set ears, and widely-spaced nipples. The neonate should be further evaluated for

   a. Klinefelter syndrome
   b. Marfan syndrome
   c. Turner syndrome

134. To ingest 120 calories/kg/day, an infant breastfeeding or receiving unfortified formula needs to ingest

   a. 3 ounces/kg/day
   b. 6 ounces/kg/day
   c. 8 ounces/kg/day

135. Which of the following drug(s) should always be included with infant resuscitation equipment?

   a. prostaglandin and epinephrine
   b. epinephrine and naloxone
   c. surfactant and naloxone

136. To reduce the risk of hemorrhagic disease after birth, a neonate should receive

   a. vitamin B9 (folic acid)
   b. vitamin C
   c. vitamin K

137. To facilitate bonding between the woman and her neonate if the woman chooses to bottle feed, the nurse should encourage the woman to

   a. maintain eye contact with the neonate
   b. hold the infant with the head higher than the body
   c. swaddle the infant tightly in a blanket

138. If a woman admitted in labor plans to relinquish her infant for adoption, the nurse should

   a. avoid any mention of adoption
   b. acknowledge the adoption plans
   c. ask the woman if she has changed her mind

139. The electrolytes that are of primary concern in the neonate are

   a. calcium, sodium, and potassium
   b. calcium, chloride, and magnesium
   c. sodium, phosphorous, and potassium

140. A neonate exposed to morphine during fetal development has episodes of high-pitched frantic crying. Comfort measures include

a. sedatives and decreased environmental stimuli
b. non-nutritive sucking and repetitive sounds
c. decreased environmental stimuli, swaddling, and rocking

141. On the APGAR scale, a good score is

a. ≥5
b. ≥7
c. ≥10

142. If, when a new mother is trying to breastfeed, the neonate latches on just to the nipple, the nurse should advise the mother to

a. use a C or U hold to gently force the nipple into the mouth
b. wait one or two minutes to see if the infant latches on correctly
c. insert a finger to break suction and start over

143. If a nursing neonate has a 5:1 suck/swallow ratio, this indicates

a. non-nutritive suckling.
b. fast but adequate suckling
c. normal suckling.

144. A neonate should no longer exhibit head lag with the pull-to-sit test by age

a. 2 weeks
b. 4 weeks
c. 4 months

145. A neonate had necrotizing enterocolitis, resulting in removal of a significant portion of the jejunum and short gut/bowel syndrome. The neonate is likely to have malabsorption of

a. fat soluble vitamins (A, D, E, K)
b. vitamin B_{12}
c. calories, proteins, carbohydrates, and fats

146. Evidence that an infant is feeding appropriately for discharge includes

a. weight gain of 15-30 grams per day
b. feeding accomplished with minimal respiratory difficulty
c. primary caregiver feeding the infant correctly at least 90% of the time

147. If a newborn begins to bob the head and bring the hands to the mouth, this may be a(n)

a. sign of neuromuscular disorder
b. feeding cue
c. indication of sleepiness

148. The pain control measure that is appropriate for a newborn that has just had a circumcision is

a. codeine
b. baby aspirin and oral sucrose
c. acetaminophen

149. The vaccination that should be routinely administered to all newborns within 24 hours of birth is

   a. hepatitis A
   b. hepatitis B
   c. hepatitis C

150. When facilitating quality improvement, the biggest barrier to implementation of changes is usually

   a. staff resistance
   b. cost constraints
   c. time constraints

151. A newborn should normally breastfeed

   a. 7-8 times in 24 hours
   b. 8-12 times in 24 hours
   c. 15-16 times in 24 hours

152. Normal term neonate skin appearance at birth should include

   a. dry peeling skin, lack of vernix, and little subcutaneous fat
   b. translucent, red, visible blood vessels and scant vernix
   c. deep cracks, no visible blood vessels, and little vernix

153. When levels of estrogen and progesterone decrease in the postpartal period, this results in increased levels of

   a. TSH
   b. prolactin
   c. T4

154. Freshly expressed human milk can be stored at room temperature for

   a. 2 hours
   b. 4 hours
   c. 6 hours

155. Following birth, an infant of a diabetic mother (IDM) is at greatest risk of hypoglycemia at

   a. 6 hours
   b. 3 to 4 hours
   c. 0.5 to 1.5 hours

156. A neonate is diagnosed with galactosemia through routine newborn metabolic screening. In order to prevent severe intellectual disability, the neonate must only receive

   a. human milk
   b. lactose-free formula
   c. iron-fortified formula

157. If a newborn develops diaper dermatitis, the initial treatment should be to

   a. apply a topical antibiotic
   b. cleanse, dry, and expose to air
   c. cleanse, dry, and apply a barrier ointment

158. Postpartum depression most often occurs at about

a. three months postpartum
b. one week postpartum
c. four weeks postpartum

159. Women who are pregnant should avoid contact with cat feces because of risk of infection with

a. parvovirus
b. *Bartonella henselae*
c. toxoplasmosis

160. Normal vital signs for a term infant who is awake but not crying are

a. HR 160, BP 70/44, RR 40
b. HR 100, BP 90/50, RR 60
c. HR 200, BP 110/70, RR 30

161. A neonate with congestive heart failure is receiving furosemide to relieve pulmonary edema. Furosemide increases the risk of

a. hyperkalemia, hyperchloremia, and hypercalcemia
b. hypokalemia, hypochloremia, and hypocalcemia
c. hypokalemia, hyperchloremia, and hypocalcemia

162. A neonate with DiGeorge syndrome (22q11.2 deletion) has severe immunocompromise as indicated by an exceptionally low

a. T-lymphocyte count
b. monocyte count
c. B-lymphocyte count

163. One of the most common causes of infant-to-infant spread of infection in hospitals is

a. antibiotic resistance
b. infant immunocompromise
c. inadequate handwashing

164. A male newborn has hypospadias. The two other most common anomalies that are often found in association with hypospadias include

a. undescended testicles and bladder exstrophy
b. inguinal hernia and undescended testicles
c. testicular torsion and inguinal hernia

165. The maternal sexually-transmitted disease that can infect the neonate and cause the multiple system disorders, including non-viral hepatitis, hepatosplenomegaly, myocarditis, palmer/plantar rash, and bone marrow failure, is

a. trichomoniasis
b. syphilis
c. chlamydia

166. Retinopathy of prematurity is associated with

    a. hypoxia

    b. congenital defect

    c. hyperoxia

167. If a mother is blood type O and the fetus type A or B, the neonate may develop

    a. hyperbilirubinemia

    b. erythroblastosis fetalis

    c. congestive heart failure

168. During the neonate's physical assessment for the Babinski reflex, stroking the lateral aspect of the sole of the foot from the heel to the ball of the foot should elicit

    a. hyperflexion (curling) of the toes

    b. hyperextension (fanning) of the toes

    c. flexion of the ankle

169. If a neonate with spina bifida exhibits slight bulging of the fontanels and distended scalp veins, this likely indicates

    a. hydrocephalus

    b. intraventricular hemorrhage

    c. normal finding

170. A female neonate with congenital adrenal hyperplasia will most likely have

    a. normal appearing genitalia

    b. both male and female gonads

    c. enlarged clitoris or male-appearing genitalia

171. If a neonate shows a sudden rapid drop of platelet count from 200,000 to 50,000 four days after birth, the most likely cause is

    a. sepsis

    b. hemorrhage

    c. hypoxia

172. If a neonate must have a transfusion with packed red blood cells, it should be given in increments of

    a. 20 to 30 mL/kg

    b. 15 to 20 mL/kg

    c. 5 to 10 mL/kg

173. The only immunoglobulin that can cross the placenta is

    a. IgA

    b. IgM

    c. IgG

174. Insensible water loss in neonates includes

    a. urination

    b. evaporated fluids

    c. gastric drainage

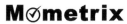

175. A mother develops mastitis and is taking antibiotics but is very uncomfortable. The mother should

    a.   avoid nursing on the affected side

    b.   use nipple guards when breastfeeding

    c.   massage the breasts in a warm shower

Answer Key and Explanations

1. A: A neonate is at risk of developing congenital varicella syndrome if the mother became infected in the first 20 weeks of pregnancy, especially from week 8 to week 20. Congenital varicella syndrome can cause a number of abnormalities of the skin, extremities, eyes, and central nervous system. Brain abnormalities may include microcephaly, hydrocephalus, cortical atrophy, enlargement of the ventricles, and damage to the sympathetic nervous system. The child may suffer intellectual disabilities and developmental delays.

2. C: Asymmetric intrauterine growth restriction is caused by problems that occur during the third trimester and typically result from problems with the function of the uterus and placenta and/or nutritional deficiency. Usually the brain and heart have normal development and the neonate has normal length but is in less than the 10th percentile for weight. The abdominal organs may be underdeveloped. The neonate will usually develop normally with adequate nutrition after birth.

3. B: If a preterm neonate has persistent episodes of apnea lasting greater than 20 seconds resulting in heart rate of 76 bpm and pallor/cyanosis, suggesting apnea of prematurity, the drug of choice to stimulate respirations is caffeine via IV or PO 10-20 mg/kg and then 5-10 mg/kg daily for maintenance. Adverse effects include gastrointestinal upset, vomiting, and bloody stools. An alternate drug is theophylline, but it may cause tachycardia and hyperglycemia. Doxapram results in decreased cerebral blood flow and is reserved for use if the other treatments are ineffective.

4. C: Nevus flammeus (port-wine stain) birthmark is an unraised demarcated red-purple lesion caused by capillaries below the epidermis. Nevus flammeus occurs most frequently on the face although it can also occur on other parts of the body. **Nevus vasculosus** (strawberry mark) is a capillary hemangioma and is a raised, demarcated dark red lesion. **Mongolian spots** are blue-black discolored areas on the buttocks and dorsal areas of dark-skinned infants, such as Asians and African Americans.

5. B: Before a heelstick to obtain a blood sample, a neonate can be provided a sucrose-dipped pacifier about 2 minutes before the procedure. The pacifier is dipped in 0.05 to 2.0 mL 12% to 24% sucrose solution (such as Sweet-Ease®); however, the pacifier must be re-dipped every two minutes. It can be dipped three additional times. Sucrose-dipped pacifiers are contraindicated for preterm infants of less than 32 weeks, severely ill neonates, and those already receiving sedation.

6. A: The most common indication for vacuum-assisted delivery of a fetus is an extended second stage of labor because longer duration correlates with increased maternal risk from trauma (hemorrhage, lacerations, chorioamnionitis). Vacuum-assisted delivery may also be utilized if the mother's health or state of exhaustion precludes normal delivery and if there is suspected fetal compromise. Contraindications include advanced cranial molding, uncertain fetal station or position, and malpresentation. Relative contraindications include preterm fetus, overlapping cranial bones, cephalopelvic disproportion, and probable macrosomia.

7. C: An important advantage of interprofessional practice is improved communication, and this in turn leads to improved patient safety. In neonatal nursing, an interprofessional team may include physician, nurse, midwife, ultrasonographer, respiratory therapist, radiologist, pharmacist, nutritionist, and breastfeeding specialist. Each has a different but equally important role in patient care. Working together collaboratively to benefit the patient leads to a better understanding of the contributions each team member provides to the group.

8. A: A mother's smoking during pregnancy places the fetus at increased risk of low birth weight and preterm birth. In addition, miscarriages and stillbirths are more common, and the fetus may exhibit tachycardia, respiratory problems, and birth defects. After birth, the child of a smoker is at increased risk of sudden infant death syndrome. The more that a pregnant woman smokes, the greater the risk, so all pregnant women should be advised to stop smoking during pregnancy. Second-hand smoke after delivery continues to pose risks to the infant.

9. B: If a pregnant woman has chlamydia, vaginal delivery of the neonate may result in eye (ophthalmia neonatorum) and lung infections, such as pneumonia. The antibiotic prophylaxis used to prevent eye infections from gonorrhea is ineffective for chlamydia infections, which are usually treated with systemic erythromycin. If the pregnant woman is untreated, there is increased risk of premature rupture of the membranes, preterm labor, and low birth weight.

10. C: An umbilical vein catheter is more appropriate than an arterial vein catheter for infusions of packed red cells, which should never be administered per an arterial line. Arterial lines are usually preferred for most other purposes, such as administration of drugs and fluids, blood gas monitoring, and monitoring of arterial blood pressure. The umbilical vein is usually easier to catheterize than the umbilical arteries. Placement of an umbilical vein catheter should be verified by echocardiography as radiographs may not provide adequate visualization.

11. A: Pregnancy-induced hypertension (also called preeclampsia or toxemia) is a disorder that develops in approximately 5% of all pregnancies. Its main feature is new onset elevated blood pressure that develops around 20 weeks of gestation, often accompanied by proteinuria though this is no longer considered a diagnostic feature. The main detrimental effect on the fetus occurs because of longstanding hypertension that leads to utero-placental vascular insufficiency, which impairs the transfer of nutrients and oxygen to the fetus, resulting in intrauterine growth restriction (IUGR). The IUGR is usually asymmetric (fetal head size is normal for gestational age). Placental abruption also occurs more frequently.

12. C: When conducting a review of the literature as part of evidence-based research, the level of evidence based on a quasi-experimental study, such as a matched case-control study, would be categorized as level III:

- Level I: Meta-analysis, randomized controlled studies.
- Level II: One or more well-designed study, may or not be randomized.
- Level III: As above.
- Level IV: Comparative non-experimental studies.
- Level V: Case reports and clinical examples but without empirical evidence.

13. B: If a neonate is exposed to repeated alarms and is exhibiting less reaction to the sound, this is an indication of habituation. Self-regulating is a self-comforting response in which the neonate may exhibit a number of different behaviors, such as sucking, moving about, or grasping hands, in order to reduce stress. An attentional response is reacting poorly to stimuli and failing to respond to comforting measures as a response to stress.

14. A: Antiretroviral medications should be given to the neonate for the first 6 weeks of life with the first dose given within the first 6-12 hours after delivery. The perinatal transmission rate is

30% in untreated HIV positive mothers, usually acquired during delivery; however, optimal treatment reduces perinatal transmission rate to as low as 1-2%. Preventive treatment includes:

- Antiviral therapy during pregnancy: A reduced viral load in the mother lessens the likelihood of prenatal transmission.
- Elective Caesarian before the amniotic membranes rupture.
- Avoidance of breastfeeding: The risk of HIV transmission with breastfeeding is 0.7% per month of breastfeeding.

15. B: If a patient has gestational diabetes but is well controlled and without complications, induction is often carried out at 38 to 39 weeks because of the increased risk of macrosomia if the pregnancy is prolonged. If there are indications for earlier delivery, then tests for fetal lung maturity should be conducted prior to induction. Many patients who required insulin during pregnancy may not require any insulin in the days after delivery because the anti-insulin factor associated with the placenta stops with placental expulsion.

16. C: Incongruent grief occurs when the mother and the father are "out of synch" in their grieving process. It may be due to the differences in how men and women grieve, or it may be because the woman typically bonds with the infant during the pregnancy, while the father bonds after the child is born. **Anticipatory grief** occurs when a child is diagnosed with a terminal illness. The parent begins to mourn over the loss of the child before he or she expires. **Delayed grief** occurs when the grieving process is postponed months to years after the loss of a child.

17. A: Children should visit the mother and infant as soon after delivery as possible. Preparation of siblings prior to the birth can decrease anxiety and sibling rivalry by helping the children feel as though they are participants and are valued. Children should be prepared for physical changes in the mother, changing family dynamics, and infant care. A parent/teacher may use dolls to demonstrate childcare and allow the children to practice holding and caring for the baby. When possible, children should have contact with an infant, such as that of a friend or family member, before delivery.

18. C: Critical congenital heart disease screening (CCHD) is carried out on the newborn through physical examination and pulse oximetry. The infant's color should be pink and heart rate at rest 110 to 160 and capillary refill time equal to or less than 3 seconds. Indications of cardiac insufficiency include change in color (pallor, circumoral cyanosis), and tachypnea. Pulse oximetry should be ≥95% with ≤3% difference between readings in the right hand and foot. If the reading is <94%, it should be retested. Readings of ≥90% are emergent and require immediate assessment by physician.

19. A: In the nonstress test (NST), fetal heart rate acceleration without movement probably indicates adequate oxygenation. A reactive (reassuring) finding includes at least 2 fetal heart rate accelerations within a 20-minute period peaking at 15 bpm or more above baseline and persisting for at least 15 seconds. These accelerations may be accompanied with movement or without, as accelerations alone are an indication fetal health. However, if fetal movement occurs without a corresponding acceleration in heart rate, this indicates fetal hypoxemia and acidosis.

20. C: If a neonate is exhibiting airway compromise, the bronchodilator that is likely to have the fewest adverse effects is levalbuterol (Xopenex®) 0.63 mg, usually administered in 1-2 puffs per MIDI twice daily. Adverse effects related to albuterol include tachycardia, irritability, GI upset, and hypokalemia. Adverse effects of levalbuterol are similar but less pronounced. Theophylline may cause tachycardia, cardiac arrhythmias, seizure activity, and irritability.

21. A: The Quad Screen includes: (1) Alpha-fetoprotein (AFP), (2) Human chorionic gonadotropin (hCG), (3) Estriol (uE³), and (4) Inhibin A (INH-A).

Disorder	AFP	hCG	uE³	INH-A
Neural tube defects	High	normal	normal	normal
Trisomy 21	Low	High	Low	High
Trisomy 18	Low	Low	Low	Low
Multiple gestation	High	High	normal	normal

22. B: If a Haitian woman states that she does not want to name her baby girl, the nurse should assume that delayed naming is a cultural norm. In fact, Haitians usually wait until after the first month to give their neonates a name. Naming holds special importance in many cultures, and names may be chosen to reflect religion, such as names chosen from the Bible or the Koran. Some Africans believe that the name may affect the child's fate. In some cultures, such as traditional Chinese, the father decides on the name.

23. A: When placing a newborn in a safety car seat, the seat should be rear facing and reclined 30 to 45 degrees (about half-way back) as this prevents the neonate's head from falling forward in a crash and blocking the airway. If the seat is reclined too far, the infant may slide backward (toward the front of the car) during a crash, injuring the head. A safety car bed may be necessary for premature infants.

24. C: Meconium testing is able to detect maternal drug use for the previous 20 weeks; however, the sample must be collected within 48 hours of birth. Urine testing detects only recent drug use (2 days after heroin and 12 hours after alcohol). Hair and nail testing can provide information about drug use during the previous 3 months and is much more sensitive than urine testing, but hair testing is more effective with curly dark hair than lighter hair. Blood testing is usually avoided because it is invasive.

25. A: With electronic fetal monitoring, an abrupt variable deceleration often indicates cord compression. It may also indicate some other acute cause of sudden decreased perfusion. Abrupt decelerations usually have a V or U shape on the monitor and may or may not occur in association with uterine contractions. The onset of the deceleration to the beginning of nadir is less than 30 seconds. The deceleration is ≥15 bpm for ≥15 seconds but <2 minutes.

26. B: The newborn hearing test that measures the integrity of the middle and inner ear and the outer hair cells of the cochlea is the otoacoustic emissions test. Otoacoustic emissions (OAE) are sounds generated by the cochlea, the inner ear structure. The audiologist conducts the OAE test by inserting a probe into the infant's external auditory canal, and stimulating the cochlea with several clicking noises. The audiologist uses a microphone to measure the evoked OAE sent off by the cochlea.

27. C: Breech presentations are present in about 3% of births and more common in preterm births, fetal abnormalities, and uterine/pelvic abnormalities. Breech positions include:

- Frank: The legs are completely extended toward the shoulders and head with the buttocks presenting.
- Full/Complete: The fetus is in flexed position with the legs flexed against the abdomen and chest as in cephalic presentation except that the fetus is reversed with the head in superior position.
- Footling: One or both legs are extended and presenting through the maternal pelvis ahead of the buttocks.

28. A: By two hours after birth, the neonate's PaO_2 should have stabilized at 80 to 95 mm Hg. Normal values include:

- Acidity/alkalinity (pH): 7.26-7.44.
- Partial pressure of carbon dioxide ($PaCO_2$): 35-45 mm Hg.
- Partial pressure of oxygen (PaO_2): >80 mg Hg.
- Bicarbonate concentration (HCO_3): 22-28 mEq/L.
- Oxygen saturation (SaO_2): >92-95%.

At birth (cord blood), the $PaCO_2$ ranges from 32-66 mm Hg and PaO_2 from 8-24 mm Hg, but these values should stabilize after the first hour as the neonate adjusts to life outside the uterus.

29. C: Because of the increased maternal blood volume during pregnancy, the maternal blood pressure often remains within normal limits even with extensive blood loss, and tachycardia may occur late as well, so often a better early indicator is a change in the fetal heart rate, either bradycardia or tachycardia, which suggests that the fetus is in distress because of the decreased oxygenation. Causes of maternal hemorrhage include placenta previa and abruptio placentae.

30. B: A pregnant patient with BP 150/100, proteinuria 0.5 g in a 24-hour specimen, normal platelet count, and normal urinary output with no complaints of pain would be classified as having mild preeclampsia. Parameters for mild preeclampsia include new onset blood pressure increase to 140-160/90-110 with or without proteinuria ≥0.3g - <2 g in 24-hour specimen (or 1+ on dipstick). Other parameters (platelets, liver enzymes, urinary output, headaches, abdominal/epigastric pain, visual disturbances, pulmonary edema, heart failure, cyanosis, and fetal growth restriction) remain within normal limits or are absent with mild preeclampsia but not with severe.

31. C: Consistent late decelerations are almost always an indication of uteroplacental insufficiency of some kind, indicating that the fetus is not adequately oxygenated. While the late deceleration is similar in appearance to an early deceleration, it begins after the uterine contraction starts and the nadir is after the contraction stops. If an occasional late deceleration occurs with variability, it is usually not cause for concern, but a consistent pattern with little or no variability and without accelerations requires immediate intervention.

32. A: During induction of labor with oxytocin, if hypertonic contractions develop, the initial response should be to immediately reduce the dosage of oxytocin or discontinue the oxytocin. Then, the primary intravenous solution should be increased and the patient repositioned into a side lying position to reduce pressure on the vena cava and aorta. In order to promote maternal oxygenation and oxygenation of the fetus, the patient should be administered oxygen at 8 to 10L/min.

33. B: The three levels of motor organization are (1) the spinal cord (which mediates automatic movement and reflexes and receives impulses from sensory neurons and sends impulses per the motor neurons to the body), (2) brain stem (which includes the medial descending systems that control body movement and antigravity reflexes and the lateral descending systems that control voluntary limb movements) and (3) the cerebral cortex (which regulates movement and controls higher cognitive and behavioral functions).

34. C: The HELLP syndrome is characterized by (H) hemolysis, (EL) elevated liver enzymes, and (LP) low platelet count. HELLP syndrome is most common in multiparous women during weeks 27 to 37 but may occur within 24 hours after delivery. Pain in the right upper quadrant related to liver dysfunction may be misdiagnosed as gastrointestinal upset or gall bladder disease. Initial symptoms are often flu-like, including headache, nausea and vomiting and visual disturbances. Mortality rates are high without promote diagnosis and treatment.

35. A: Conditions associated with oligohydramnios (<500 mL) include urinary tract anomalies. After week 20 of gestation, most amniotic fluid is produced by fetal urine, so if urine production is inadequate, the volume decreases. Oligohydramnios can lead to pressure deformities (such as club foot), pulmonary hypoplasia, and compression of the umbilical cord. Chromosomal abnormalities (trisomy 21, 18, and 13) and obstructional lesions of the GI tract are associated with polyhydramnios (>500 mL).

36. B: If a neonate is often restless and sleeps about 12 out of 24 hours, this amount of sleep is inadequate and assessment should be carried out to determine the reason. Neonates normally sleep about 70% to 80% of the time initially (16-19 out of 24 hours), waking every 1 to 3 hours to nurse or feed and then falling back asleep. Wake times extend slowly as the infant grows. Initially the neonate's sleeping time during the day and nighttime are about the same, but by 8 to 12 weeks, the infant may begin sleeping longer during the night.

37. A: A normal biophysical score is 10 (score of 2 on 5 different measures). A score of 8 with normal volume of amniotic fluid suggests very little risk to the fetus and no intervention is required. If, however, the amniotic fluid volume were abnormal, this would suggest chronic asphyxia and increased rate of perinatal mortality with a week, so birth should be induced. A score of 6 indicates possible asphyxia, 4 probably asphyxia, 2 almost certain asphyxia, and 0 certain asphyxia.

38. C: If a neonate who was exposed to maternal opioid drugs prenatally is undergoing neonatal abstinence syndrome with NAS score of 9 three times consecutively (Finnegan scale), indicting the need for medical treatment, the drug of choice is generally diluted tincture of opium although some may use morphine or methadone. Second line drugs include phenobarbital and clonidine for neonates who do not respond adequately to opioids.

39. A: Within 2 to 3 hours of birth, a newborn's temperature should stabilize at 36.5 to 37° C (97.7 to 98.6° F). After birth, a newborn's temperature can fall quite rapidly when exposed to environmental air, which is far cooler than intrauterine temperatures. The newborn may lose up to 0.3° C (0.5° F) every minute, up to about 3° C (5.4° F), especially if subjected to cold stress. The newborn should be immediately placed on the mother's body or under a radiant warmer when examined and should be dried of amniotic fluid to prevent heat loss from evaporation.

40. A: If a newborn with myelomeningocele has passed no urine in more than 24 hours, the most likely reason is neurogenic bladder, a common finding with this form of neural tube defect. If neurogenic bladder is suspected, the newborn should undergo renal ultrasound and urodynamic studies. Treatment may include medications, Credé massage (not usually effective with myelodysplasia), and clean intermittent catheterization to prevent nephrosis and permanent kidney damage. Surgical intervention, such as creating a urinary diversion, may promote later independence.

41. B: A new mother should be advised that, by day 4 after birth, a neonate should urinate approximately 6 times daily. Most neonates urinate within 12 to 24 hours of birth and then urinate one or two times a day during the first 2 days; but, by day four, neonates should urinate approximately 6 times daily. The kidneys produce a normal urinary output of 2 to 5 mL/kg per hour in a neonate. Neonates are prone to acidosis because the kidneys are less able to excrete bicarbonate than older children and adults.

42. C: The most common complication of multiple births is preterm birth, which occurs in 6 out of 10 twin births and almost all triplets or greater multiple births. The multiples also have double the risk of birth defects as singletons. Twin-to-twin transfusion syndrome occurs with about 15% of identical twins that share a placenta. Other complications include increased rate of miscarriage of all or part of the fetuses. The mother is at increased risk for iron-deficiency anemia and gestational hypertension.

43. B: Pathological jaundice is usually evident within the first 24 hours after birth while physiological jaundice, which occurs in up to 80% of neonates, is evident between 24 and 48 hours after birth. Pathological jaundice may result in rapid increase of total serum bilirubin and is diagnosed at 12.9 mg/dL in a full-term infant and 15 mg/dL in a preterm infant. Conditions that result in accelerated breakdown of red blood cells, such as polycythemia, birth trauma, and Rh incompatibility increase bilirubin levels.

44. A: On day one of birth for a term infant, the normal blood glucose level should be 40 to 60 mg/dL (2.2 to 3.3 mmol/L), increasing to 50 to 80 mg/dL (2.8 to 4.4 mmol/L) by day 2. Because capillary screening is less accurate than blood glucose, a low value should be verified by laboratory analysis. Typically, an infant is fed if values are 40 to 45 mg/dL (2.2 to 2.5 mmol/L) or less, especially with signs of hypoglycemia, and then the value rechecked 30 to 60 minutes after feedings until it remains above 50 mg/dL (2.8 mmol/L) twice.

45. A: Parents should be taught to place a neonate on the back when the neonate is sleeping and unattended at all times to decrease the risk of sudden infant death syndrome (SIDS). Ideally, the baby should sleep in the same room with a parent for the first year, but in a separate crib on a firm mattress with a fitted sheet but no blankets, toys, or other bedding. The slats of the crib must be no more than 6 cm apart to prevent the neonate from getting the head caught between the slats.

46. B: Kangaroo Care consists of placing the infant in minimal clothing in an upright position on the mother's bare chest between her breasts to allow for skin-to-skin contact. Benefits to the neonate include better regulation of vital signs, reduced stress, decreased episodes of apnea, increased weight gain, fewer infections, and enhanced neonate-maternal bonding. Benefits to the mother include enhanced bonding, increased milk production, and increased confidence in providing infant care.

47. C: Autonomy is the ethical principle that the individual has the right to make decisions about her own care, based on informed consent and understanding of risks and benefits. **Beneficence** is an ethical principle that involves performing actions that are for the purpose of benefitting another person. **Nonmaleficence** is an ethical principle that means healthcare workers should provide care in a manner that does not cause direct intentional harm to the patient.

48. B: On the New Ballard Score for assessment of gestational age, a score of zero (0) indicates 24 weeks, the gestational age at which a fetus is considered viable. Scores range from -10 (20 weeks) to 50 (44 weeks) with each increase of 5 points on the scale indicating 2 additional weeks of gestation, so a score of +5 is equal to 26 weeks. The New Ballard Sore assesses 6 measures of neuromuscular maturity (posture, square window, arm recoil, popliteal angle, scarf sign, and heel to ear) and 6 measures of physical maturity (skin, lanugo, plantar surface, breast, eye/ear, genitals).

49. B: The most common reason for elevated bilirubin levels in a breastfed infant (breastfeeding jaundice) within a week of birth is inadequate intake of human milk. If the child does not nurse adequately because of excessive sleepiness, poor sucking, or infrequent nursing, the child may not ingest enough colostrum to benefit from its laxative effect, which helps to eliminate meconium, which is high in bilirubin. The mother may need assistance with breastfeeding to increase the neonate's intake and the production of milk.

50. C: Fetal bradycardia with variable decelerations during uterine contractions may indicate prolapsed cord. In some cases, the cord may be seen protruding from the vagina, especially after rupture of the membranes if the presenting part is high, or felt on digital exam. Immediate action is required to prevent fetal hypoxia. The patient is placed in modified Sims' or knee chest position and the examiner inserts fingers into the vagina to hold the presenting cord off of the cord while awaiting emergent treatment, such as Caesarean.

51. A: RHuEPO is indicated to stimulate erythropoiesis in phlebotomy-related AOP. Infants with signs of hypoxemia (poor feeding, tachypnea, tachycardia, pallor) may require transfusions. AOP represents a pathologic exaggeration of the normal decrease in hematocrit that occurs in every newborn. Other causes include:

- Decreased RBC production because the premature neonate's response to erythropoietin (EPO), the main stimulus for RBC production, has not matured. Lowest Hgb levels are usually at 2-3 months of age.
- Premature RBCs have a shortened lifespan when compared to the full-term neonate's because of decreased levels of intracellular ATP and enzyme activity.

52. B: Placing the newborn infant against the mother's bare skin helps to reduce conductive heat loss, which occurs when the neonate contacts objects with lower temperature than the neonate's skin. Drying the neonate immediately helps prevent evaporative heat loss and providing a warm environment, free of drafts, helps prevent convective heat loss. Placing the child into a radiant warmer transfers heat from the warmer to the neonate through radiation.

53. A: If a neonate has been diagnosed with craniotabes because of a softened area of skull in the posterior occipital area, the most likely treatment is observation only because most cases are benign. Craniotabes are common (in up to 30% of newborns) and usually resolve within the first 4 weeks of life. However, the infant should be carefully examined for indications of disease-related causes of craniotabes, including other conditions that effect bone growth or hardness, such as rickets, syphilis, marasmus, or osteogenesis imperfecta.

54. B: With acute respiratory distress syndrome (ARDS) in the neonate, the goal of therapy is to maintain oxygen saturation >90%. If ARDS is mild, oxygen administration per nasal prongs or mask may be adequate, but if levels fall <90% then endotracheal intubation with mechanical ventilation or high-frequency oscillatory ventilation may be indicated. ARDS is characterized by tachypnea, crackling rales, decreased lung volume, cyanosis, hypotension, and tachycardia. In the early stages, respiratory alkalosis is common but later develops into hypercarbia and respiratory acidosis.

55. C: Early onset sepsis most often is characterized by pneumonia and late onset by bacteremia and/or meningitis. Neonatal sepsis is a particular risk for preterm infants <1000 g and may be associated with a wide range of pathogens, both bacterial and viral. Early onset (≤72 hours) is usually related to maternal transmission and late onset (4 to 90 days) to invasive devices. Septic pneumonia usually presents with tachypnea, sternal retraction, grunting respirations, cyanosis, and apneic periods.

56. B: Steps in treatment of hypothermia:

1. Increase the air temperature by approximately 1°C every hour until the infant's temperature is normal and stable.
2. Determine if the cause of hypothermia is from an abnormal physiological process in the infant or from environmental conditions.
3. Avoid rewarming the infant too rapidly because rapid rewarming may result in apnea or hypotension. Maintain the ambient temperature at 1 to 1.5°C higher than the infant's temperature.
4. Warm IV fluids with a blood-warming device prior to infusion.
5. Closely monitor the infant's blood glucose levels, vital signs, and urinary output.

57. C: A contrast enema is used to confirm a diagnosis of meconium plug syndrome and helps differentiate that from other causes of intestinal obstruction. The contrast enema also is often therapeutic and helps the plug to pass. Meconium plug syndrome usually occurs in full term infants, infants of diabetic mothers, or infants with hypermagnesemia. A small percentage of infants initially identified as having meconium plug syndrome (5 to 10%) have Hirschsprung disease. The cause of meconium plug syndrome is thought to be immaturity of the ganglion cells of the colon.

58. B: Caput succedaneum is edema of the fetal scalp resulting from pressure of the head against the cervix (or from suction of vacuum-assisted delivery). The swelling crosses suture lines and is usually soft and resolves within the first 12 hours after delivery. **Cephalohematoma** is bleeding between the periosteum and the skull. The swelling is usually firm, most commonly over parietal areas, and does not cross suture lines. **Molding** is an overlapping of cranial bones at suture lines. This condition usually resolves within a week.

59. C: The head circumference is usually about 2 cm greater than the chest circumference, so the head circumference should be about 36 cm. Expected findings in a term neonate is the following:

Head	Disproportionately large for body.
Body	Long with prominent abdomen and narrow hips.
Extremities	Short and in flexed position. (Feet usually dorsiflexed after breech birth.) Hands clenched.
Neck	Short and chin resting on chest
Weight	2500-4000 g (average about 3400). Physiologic weight loss is 5-10% for full term and 15% for preterm.
Length	45-55 cm (average 50 cm).
Head circumference	32-38 cm (usually 2 cm greater than chest circumference)
Chest circumference	Chest rounded and 30-36 cm

60. A: While the neonate's bilirubin is elevated (normal range 3.4 to 11.5 mg/dL at 1 to 2 days), only continued observation and jaundice assessment is indicated at this time. Physiologic hyperbilirubinemia is common in newborns and usually benign, resulting from immature hepatic function and increased RBC hemolysis. Infants have larger red blood cells with a shorter life than adults, leading to more RBC destruction and resulting in an increased load of serum bilirubin, which the liver of the newborn cannot handle. Onset is usually within 24 to 48 hours, peaking in 72 hours for full term or 5 days for preterm infants and declining within a week. Phototherapy is the indicated treatment for total serum bilirubin ≥18 mg/dL for those at medium risk.

61. C: Swaddling a neonate exposed to cocaine and eliminating as much environmental noise and excessive light as possible can reduce stimulation and relieve symptoms. Medications are rarely required to control symptoms. Hypertonia may last ≤2 years. Head circumference may be smaller for the first 2 years as well although the infant usually attains normal weight and height by the end of the first year.

62. B: Umbilical cord blood gas testing, preferably arterial, should be done ≤60 minutes of birth for infants who are at risk or depressed to determine pH and acid-base balance. Testing is most applicable to infants with low APGAR scores (0-3) persisting for ≥5 minutes.

Normal cord blood values

	Venous	Arterial
pH	7.25 to 7.35	7.28
PO₂	28-32 mm Hg.	16-20 mm Hg.
PCO₂	40-50 mm Hg.	40-50 mm Hg.
Base excess	0 to 5 mEq/L	0-10 mEq/L

63. A: Erythema toxicum is a skin eruption of erythematous papules, vesicles, and sometimes pustules. Erythema toxicum is essentially benign and occurs in ≥50% of newborns. It is a generalized rash everywhere except the palms and soles of the feet, usually occurring 2-3 days after birth. **Neonatal pustular melanosis** is a benign rash (vesicles and macules) but not associated with erythema. **Cutis marmorata** is a disorder in which the infant's skin mottles or marbles when exposed to cold because the superficial blood vessels dilate and contract at the same time.

64. A: Autosomal recessive: Recurrence is 25% for each pregnancy and 50% risk of the child becoming a carrier. **Autosomal dominant:** Recurrence risk is 50%, but there is no carrier state. **X-linked recessive:** Recurrence risk is 50% for affected sons and 50% risk of daughters becoming carriers. Affected sons do not pass the disorder to sons, but all daughters become carriers. **X-linked dominant:** Father passes the disorder to 100% of daughters but no sons. Mother passes the trait to 50% of sons and 50% of daughters, but daughters are usually unaffected.

65. C: Cystic fibrosis is a congenital disease associated with thick collection of mucous in the lungs and intestines. Up to a fifth of children born with cystic fibrosis has meconium ileus. Meconium ileus is obstruction of the ileum with inspissated (thick) mucilaginous meconium that clings to the side of the narrowed lumen of the intestine and forms hard pellets (usually the first clinical sign of cystic fibrosis). The mucus interferes with absorption of fat, protein, carbohydrates, and other nutrients, leading to malabsorption syndromes.

66. A: Jitteriness is the likely cause and is distinct from **shuddering**, a 10-15 second period of fast tremors that may recur ≤100 times daily. Both jitteriness and shuddering are benign findings.

Seizures indicate that there is an abnormality of the central nervous system and are differentiated by their associated abnormal movements:

- Subtle: Feet pedaling, chewing, apnea, eye movements, or blank stare.
- Tonic: Tonic flexion or extension of the limbs, focal (one limb) or generalized.
- Clonic: Slow, clonic movements (1-3 per second), often in one extremity or one side of the body.
- Myoclonic: Focal, multi-focal, or generalized, with rapid jerking movements of the extremities.

67. B: A glucose bolus-associated occurrence of acute hypoglycemia can arise if a glucose bolus is given and not followed up with a continuous infusion because the body will produce more insulin to cover the bolus which will then start to use glucose stores as soon as the bolus stops. To prevent this, a steady infusion should be continued for a time period that is sufficient for the infant's insulin production to stabilize. Bedside tests for hypoglycemia with reagent sticks may overestimate hypoglycemia and should be confirmed with a serum level.

68. A: Café au lait spots (CAL) are flat skin lesions with increased melanin content and regular or irregular borders. If the CAL spots are faint, one can use a Wood lamp to make them easier to see. Fewer than 3 café au lait spots have no clinical significance. However, 6 or more café au lait spots with a diameter larger than 5 mm occur in 95% of patients with neurofibromatosis type 1 (NF1), a disorder of chromosome 17. Lisch nodules on the child's iris and Crowe's sign (freckles on the axilla and inguinal area) corroborate the diagnosis of NF1.

69. B: Intravenous acyclovir is given to infants exposed to herpes virus. Most vertical transmissions occur when the neonate travels through a colonized birth canal. The transmission rate from women with a primary HSV infection is approximately 50%, while the transmission rate is 1-2% if the infection is a recurrence of HSV. Signs of a neonatal infection with HSV include:

- Skin, eye, and mucous membrane blistering at 10-12 days of life.
- Disseminated disease may spread to multiple organs, leading to pneumonitis, hepatitis, and intravascular coagulation.
- Encephalitis may be the only presentation, with signs of lethargy, irritability, poor feeding, and seizures.

70. C: Sensorineural hearing loss occurs when the cochlea is impaired or damaged by a genetic syndrome, *in utero* infections like rubella, postnatal meningitis, or ototoxic medication (such as aminoglycoside antibiotics or the diuretic furosemide). **Conductive** hearing loss occurs from an abnormality in the sound conduction system in the outer and middle ears (external ear canal, tympanic membrane, and auditory ossicles). **Central** hearing loss is rare and occurs when defects or damage of the auditory nervous pathway or auditory brain centers are present in infants with kernicterus, episodes of hypoxia, or intraventricular hemorrhage.

71. A: Asymmetry in gluteal and thigh creases in a neonate may indicate developmental hip dysplasia, which is hip instability that results from the femoral head and acetabulum being misaligned. The condition worsens as the child ages. Tests to identify developmental hip dysplasia include:

- Ortolani: Positive findings occur when applying pressure at the head of the femur with hips in flexed position causes posterior subluxation.
- Barlow: Positive findings occur when hips are rotated through range of motion and an audible click is heard at abduction because the femoral head slips out of place.

72. B: If on auscultation of the neonate's heart sounds, the S1 sound, heard as the mitral and tricuspid valves close, is louder than normal, this may be an indication of ventricular septal defect, patent ductus arteriosus, or tetralogy of Fallot. The louder sound indicates that the cardiac output and blood flow are higher than normal. If the S1 sound is quieter than normal, this may indicate congestive heart failure or myocarditis.

73. C: When assessing the plantar grasp reflex in a neonate, a normal response is flexion of the toes. The reflex is elicited by firmly touching the area beneath the toes. This should cause the toes to immediately flex and curl toward the bottom of the foot, similar to the palmar grasp reflex in the hand. However, if the lateral sole is stroked, this will elicit a primitive Babinski reflex in the neonate, and the toes will flare and extend while the great toe dorsiflexes.

74. B: If meconium was detected in the amniotic fluid during delivery of a neonate and, at birth, the infant is hypotonic and respirations are depressed the infant should be placed on a radiant warmer and the mouth cleared of secretions with a bulb syringe. Endo-tracheal suctioning is no longer advised. Only if the neonate's respiratory status does not improve or the neonate's heart rate falls to below 100 bpm is positive pressure ventilation is indicated.

75. C: All HIV-exposed neonates whose mothers took antiretroviral drugs during pregnancy should receive HIV prophylaxis as soon as possible after birth (within 6 to 12 hours), with zidovudine, usually for 6 weeks although a 4-week course may be given if the mother had adequate viral suppression with antiretrovirals during pregnancy. Dosage is determined by the neonate's weight and weeks of gestation at birth. If the mother was not treated with antiretroviral drugs during pregnancy, then the neonate should receive both zidovudine and nevirapine.

76. A: Inhaled nitrous oxide (iNO) may be used as an inhaled pulmonary vasodilator for neonates with persistent pulmonary hypertension of the newborn (PPHN), which is sometimes a complication of meconium aspiration syndrome. iNO is used to treat PPHN in neonates without congenital heart disease and with mean airway pressure of 12-15 cmH$_2$O, decreased PaO$_2$, and pH >7.40 despite treatments and adequate ventilation. Treatment with conventional therapy (such as pressor/inotropics) should continue. INO combines with hemoglobin, which inactivates the NO and forms methemoglobin, so methemoglobin levels must be monitored frequently.

77. C: Following birth, damage to the neonate's upper brachial plexus (C5 to C7) is likely to result in Erb's palsy, which affects both the upper arm and the forearm. Movement is diminished or absent with the arm extended at the side and the forearm prone. Brachial plexus injury is associated with macrosomia, breech presentation, and shoulder dystocia. In most cases, recovery occurs within 3 to 6 months, but some infants may require surgical repair although prognosis is poor for surgical intervention. Pseudoparalysis (lack of movement because of fracture) may be misdiagnosed as brachial plexus injury.

78. B: If a neonate that suffered birth trauma with hypoxemia developed firm reddened circumscribed nodules in fatty areas of the body about 7 days after birth and is diagnosed with fat necrosis, the electrolyte that should be monitored is calcium because calcium is released as part of the healing process and may result in hypercalcemia. Medications, such as furosemide, steroids, or bisphosphonates may be indicated to treat hypercalcemia. However, lesions usually heal with no problem.

79. C: If a neonate's cardiac status appeared normal at birth but 48 hours later the neonate experiences a precipitous drop in circulation to the lower body, the likely congenital heart defect is coarctation of the aorta, which is a stricture of the aorta, proximal to the ductus arteriosus intersection. As the heart tries to pump the blood past the stricture, the blood pressure to the head and upper extremities increases decreasing blood pressure and circulation to the lower body and extremities. Symptoms may not occur until the ductus arteriosus closes, causing sudden loss of blood supply to the lower body.

80. A: Necrotizing enterocolitis in a preterm infant is usually caused by ischemic bowel. If the neonate has episodes of hypoxia, oxygen is shunted to the heart and lungs and other organs, such as the intestines, may become hypoxic. If oxygenation is inadequate, areas of necrosis occur, and this interferes with peristalsis, so stool begins to build up. Sepsis may also occur, putting the neonate at grave risk.

81. C: If a neonate has a patent ductus arteriosus, the usual initial treatment is indomethacin. If given within 10 days of birth, the medication closes about 80% of defects. Patent ductus arteriosus (PDA) occurs when the ductus arteriosus that connects the pulmonary artery and aorta fails to close after birth. This results in left to right shunting of blood from the aorta back to the pulmonary artery, increasing the blood flow to the lungs and causing an increase in pulmonary hypertension that can result in damage to the lung tissue.

82. B: Most neonates pass the first meconium within 24 hours of birth (although some may take up to 48 hours). The first meconium is thick, dark and tarry in consistency. Transitions stools for the next few days may range in color from brown to green. After that, stools of breastfed babies are yellow-gold in color and mushy consistency while those of formula-fed babies are pale yellow in color and pasty in consistency. Frequency varies with breastfed babies passing stools less frequently (because of low residue in human milk) than formula fed babies, who should have at least one stool daily.

83. A: If bloody mucoid discharge ("pseudomenstruation") is noted in a newborn's vaginal area, this is a normal finding. Vernix caseosa (white, cheesy discharge) may also be evident between the labia. The labia majora should surround the labia minor, touch and completely cover the clitoris in a full-term infant. A hymenal tag may be evident. If any stool is noted in the newborn's vagina, this may be an indication of a rectovaginal fistula. With a breech birth, the genital area may be ecchymotic and edematous.

84. B: Preterm infants are at risk of hyperkalemia primary because of potassium shift. The newborn's potassium level reflects that of the mother, but potassium levels rise after birth because potassium shifts from the intracellular space to the extracellular, especially in preterm infants. If the kidneys function adequately, the potassium levels should fall to normal within a few days. Neonatal potassium values:

- Normal value: 3.7 to 5.9 mEq/L.
- Hyperkalemia: >6 mEq/L. Critical value: >6.5 mEq/L.
- Hypokalemia: <3.5 mEq/L. Critical value: <2.5 mEq/L.

85. C: On examination, a newborn is found to have a scrotal mass that is soft and painless and does not change in size but transilluminates, probably indicating a hydrocele, which is a collection of fluid in the scrotum. If the hydrocele is noncommunicating (the opening to the sac is closed), then the fluid will usually absorb slowly over about 12 months. However, if the sac is communicating (the sac is open), fluid can flow into the abdomen and back, so the size of the hydrocele may vary. Surgical repair may be indicated if the hydrocele persists beyond 12 months or causes pain.

86. A: Small urate crystals ("brick dust spots") found in the urine of a newborn are a sign of immature renal function. The crystals may be present in the newborn's urine soon after birth because the kidneys are not efficient at filtering wastes or reabsorbing liquid. The crystals usually disappear within a few days. The newborn's infant may also have small amounts of protein and glucose during the first few days. After birth, the newborn's bladder capacity is 6 to 44 mL, and urinary output for the first 2 days is usually only about 15 mL total.

87. C: Newborns tend to regurgitate after feeding because the gastroesophageal sphincter is immature and doesn't close adequately, allowing gastric contents to reflux up the esophagus. Additionally, the newborn's stomach capacity is quite small, only about 6 mL/kg at birth, but the stomach expands to hold about 90 mL fluid by the end of the first week. With a small stomach, if gas builds up in the stomach, regurgitation is more likely to occur, so newborns should be burped with both breastfeeding and bottle-feeding. Projectile vomiting is abnormal.

88. C: If a newborn has metatarsus adductus ("toeing in") of 20 degrees in both feet, the likely treatment is serial long-leg casting. Metatarsus adductus is the most common congenital disorder of the feet and results in a convex curve with the forefoot turned inward at the tarsometatarsal joint. The abnormality may result from oligohydramnios or position in the uterus. If the curvature is less than 15 degrees, it usually corrects with stretching exercises, but with curvature of more than 15 degrees, serial casting is usually required.

89. B: If a 7-day-old newborn begins crying frantically and exhibits scrotal swelling and negative cremasteric reflex, the most likely cause is testicular torsion. Other congenital abnormalities may be present as well. Undescended testes are likely to twist when descending, so torsion at 7 to 10 days is common. The torsion must be relieved within 6 hours to prevent permanent damage. Torsion may be relieved manually or surgically although the torsion may recur if the testis is not sutured into correct position.

90. C: Transient tachypnea of the newborn (TTN) occurs because of fluid in the lungs not adequately absorbed. The infant may show signs of respiratory distress—dyspnea, sternal retraction, expiratory grunt, and nasal flaring—within 36 hours of birth, but the condition usually resolves spontaneously within 3 days. The infant is usually provided supportive care, including oxygen if the oxygen saturation level falls and IV fluids or NG feedings if the respirations are so rapid the infant is unable to take oral fluids without risk of aspiration.

91. A: An increased risk factor for pneumothorax in the newborn is caused by meconium aspiration. Signs and symptoms include increasing dyspnea with tachypnea and chest wall retractions. Breath sounds are absent on the side with the pneumothorax, and paradoxical chest movements may be evident. The newborn may develop bradycardia and cyanosis. Treatment is needle aspiration in most cases although chest tubes may need to be inserted if cardiac arrest or pleural effusion occurs. Treatment of the underlying cause is essential.

92. C: The type of seizures that are the most common in newborns is tonic seizures. The seizures may involve tonic flexion or extension of the extremities and may include one side or both. Tonic seizures are most common in preterm newborns while subtle (feet pedaling, chewing, apnea, eye movements, staring) and clonic seizures are more common in full-term. Treatment may include glucose 10% solution if seizures are related to hypoglycemia. Phenobarbital is the initial anti-seizure drug of choice.

93. B: Two weeks after birth, a newborn develops bulging fontanels, bradycardia, hypotension, and abnormal dolls-eye reflex, suggesting subdural hemorrhage, which is bleeding between the dura and the cerebrum. Subdural hemorrhage tends to develop slowly, so symptoms are often delayed, but subdural hematoma can occur over time. If the bleeding is acute and rapid, the prognosis is poor. Subdural hemorrhage is a common birth trauma, especially if the newborn has a large head or if there is a malpresentation. Treatment for subdural hemorrhage may include subdural taps or evacuation of the hematoma.

94. A: The purpose of a partial exchange transfusion for a newborn with polycythemia is to lower the hematocrit to 55 to 60%. Aliquots (no more than 5 mL at a time) of the newborn's blood are replaced with normal saline. Polycythemia is a hematocrit greater than 65%. The partial exchange transfusion is given if the newborn's hematocrit is 65% or higher with symptoms or if it is 70% with or without symptoms.

95. C: If a breastfeeding mother develops painful cracked nipples, the most likely cause is improper latching on. This is especially likely to occur if the infant is latching on only to the nipple and does not have the mouth about the areola. Other causes may include fungal infection (mouth thrush) passed from infant to mother and using excessive suction with a breast pump. The woman should review latching on procedures and be advised to rotate the neonate's feeding positions.

96. B: Grade III. Intraventricular hemorrhage classifications:

Grade I	Hemorrhage limited to the germinal matrix (subependymal region).	Mild (5% Death rate; 5% motor or cognitive impairment).
Grade II	Hemorrhage extends 10%-40% into the lateral ventricles on sagittal view, but has not dilated them significantly.	Moderate (10% Death rate; 30%-40% motor or cognitive impairment).
Grade III	Hemorrhage extends 50% or more into the lateral ventricles with significant ventricular dilation.	Severe (27%-50% Death rate; 35% motor or cognitive impairment).
Grade IV	Hemorrhage extends into brain tissue.	Periventricular hemorrhagic infarction (80% Death rate; 90% motor or cognitive impairment).

97. A: A newborn's hemoglobin from cord blood should be approximately 16.8 g/dL (168 mmol/L) and otherwise 17 to 18 g/dL (170 to 180 mmol/L). Newborns have higher levels of hemoglobin and hematocrit than adults, but these levels usually peak at about 2 hours after birth. Levels have usually fallen within a week of birth because of exposure to increased environmental oxygen. During gestation, the fetus has primarily fetal hemoglobin, which carries 20% to 50% more oxygen than adult hemoglobin, but the hemoglobin begins to be replaced later in development with adult hemoglobin, and this process continues after birth.

98. C: if a neonate has abdominal distention, bilious vomiting, diarrhea with bloody stools, tachycardia, tachypnea, and cycles of cramping pain every 15 to 30 minutes, these symptoms are consistent with a malrotation defect and volvulus, a twisted bowel that impairs circulation to that section of the bowel and can lead to bowel infarction. Treatment includes emergent surgical repair. Postoperatively, the child may begin with TPN and progress to enteral feedings during healing.

99. A: A scrotal mass that may be reduced with gentle pressure is likely an inguinal hernia. An inguinal hernia occurs when a loop of bowel or an ovary extends through the inguinal canal. Unless it incarcerates, the palpable mass is usually not painful; however, surgical repair is necessary to prevent recurrence, as the opening does not heal spontaneously. The mass may be more evident when the infant cries or strains. Hernia repair is one of the most common pediatric surgeries.

100. B: Micrognathia (small chin) may indicate an alcohol-related birth defect (AKA fetal alcohol syndrome). Other physical abnormalities may include lack of philtrum, microcephaly, cardiac, bone, and renal abnormalities, and vision and hearing impairment. The infant may sleep poorly and have difficulty sucking adequately. Over time the child may exhibit low body weight and short height as well as behavioral and cognitive impairment, speech and language delays. Treatment is supportive and often includes intervention from social services.

101. C: If a mother had previous breast reduction surgery and wants to breastfeed her neonate but her milk supply remains at about 75% of normal production, the most effective solution is to utilize a nursing supplementation system that allows the infant to nurse while the infants is receiving a supplement through a small catheter placed alongside the nipple so that the baby latches onto both the nipple and the catheter. Various systems are commercially available. Supplementation may be with formula or donor milk.

102. A: If natal teeth are noted on the newborn's physical examination, further evaluation is necessary as natal teeth are often an indication of other abnormalities. The teeth should be carefully assessed for stability by a pediatric dentist and should be removed if they are loose in order to reduce the risk of aspiration. Natal teeth are often poorly formed and loose. Natal teeth may be associated with cleft lip/palate and a number of different rare syndromes, including Meckel-Gruber, Ellis-van Creveld, and Jackson-Lawler.

103. B: If a woman was infected with Zika virus at some point during her pregnancy, the fetus is at risk for microcephaly. Zika virus is transmitted by mosquitoes and is endemic in many tropical areas, such as in Mexico, Central America, and South America. Women who have traveled to these areas during pregnancy or whose partner has done so are especially at risk. Pregnant women are advised to avoid travel in areas where Zika virus is common. Zika infections are often asymptomatic or relatively mild with fever, rash, joint pain, and conjunctivitis.

104. B: If a neonate has developed gastroesophageal reflux disease, regurgitating frequently after feeding, and the mother has been told to hold the infants at a 45-60° angle for breastfeeding, after feeding, the infant should be held upright in the arms for 30 minutes. The mother should avoid bouncing or jiggling the neonate for at least an hour. While prone position reduces reflux, it should be used only when the neonate is awake because of the risk of SIDS. Placing the neonate in an infant seat after feeding should be avoided as this may result in increased abdominal pressure.

105. C: Conductive heat loss occurs when a newborn is placed on a cold scale. Heat spreads to the colder surface. **Evaporative** heat loss occurs when fluid is converted to vapor, such as may occur if the infant remains wet with amniotic fluid that air dries, resulting in insensible water loss. **Convective** heat loss occurs when heat is lost to cooler air currents, such as if a newborn is in a draft. **Radiative** heat loss occurs when heat transfers between objects that aren't in direct contact, such as heat transfer to the walls of an incubator.

106. A: An infant is classified as large for gestational age (LGA) if the weight is above the 90th percentile for the infant's gestation. The average newborn weighs about 7 pounds (3.2 kg). A newborn may be LGA because of genetics or because the mother gained excess weight during pregnancy. Most LGA are born at term or post-term. The majority of newborns who are LGA are born to diabetic mothers. LGA fetuses are at risk for birth trauma and may require Caesarean for delivery.

107. A: During assessment of the Moro ("startle") reflex, a normal response is for the infant to extend the arms and flex the legs. The Moro reflex is assessed by slightly lifting the infant's body and head and mimicking a release that allows the head to fall back but not touch the surface underneath. This action should startle the infant and may cause the infant to cry. As the infant relaxes, the limbs move back into flexed position. The Moro reflex usually persists for 3 to 4 months.

108. B: If a newborn has been breastfeeding readily and urinating but has abdominal distention and no passage of stool for 36 hours after birth, the newborn should be assessed for imperforate anus. In some cases, such as with low and intermediate anomalies, an anal dimple is present and may have been mistaken for an anus. Low and intermediate anomalies usually require excision of the anus and minimal surgical intervention, but higher anomalies may require a colostomy and later reconstructive surgery.

109. C: If a neonate is born with gastroschisis (stomach and intestines herniating through an opening in the abdominal wall) the exposed organs should be immediately covered with moist gauze dressings and wrapped in plastic (around the neonate's body) to secure and prevent further fluid loss and hypothermia. The infant must be maintained in supine position to prevent intestinal ischemia. Surgery is usually done within 2 to 4 hours of delivery.

110. A: If a neonate has the characteristic physical differences associated with trisomy 21 (Down syndrome)—preterm birth; small size; short, round head with flat occiput; epicanthal folds; flat face; tongue protruding; hypotonia; and short fingers and square hands with single palmar simian creases—the neonate should be further evaluated for congenital heart disease. Up to 50% of neonates with trisomy 21 also have congenital heart disease, and early diagnosis and treatment is critical. Common disorders include AV septal defects, VS defects, AS defects, PDA, and other complex cardiac disorders.

111. C: If a newborn that has been circumcised urinates or defecates, the area should be cleansed with warm water only, as soap and ingredients in the baby wipes may cause irritation and discomfort. Diapers should be changed promptly. Petrolatum jelly or gauze may be applied to the incisional areas for about 4 days. The surgical area is often swollen and red and small amounts of bleeding are common for the first 24 hours.

112. A: If the newborn's color is good when the mouth is open but becomes cyanotic when the mouth is closed, this may indicate choanal atresia. This may be noted if trying without success to pass a suctioning tube through the nares. Newborns are obligate nasal breathers and may show no symptoms if only one side is affected but if the condition is bilateral, the infant may exhibit respiratory distress and cyanosis that are alleviated by crying. The infant may require intubation and ventilation as an emergent treatment, but bilateral choanal atresia requires surgical perforation of the atresia.

113. B: Screening of all pregnant women around 36 weeks of gestation followed by antibiotic treatment of the infected mother for at least 4 hours during labor can prevent neonatal infection with Group B *Streptococcus*. If the mother has not received the recommended treatment, the infant may be treated with IV ampicillin and gentamicin for 10 to 14 days. If treatment is ineffective, the infant with a GBS infection that manifests in the first 24 hours after birth may develop pneumonia and/or meningitis, respiratory distress, floppiness, poor feeding, tachycardia, shock and seizures. Late onset infections may be more severe.

114. A: The most likely treatment for a newborn that suffered a right clavicular fracture during a breech birth is arm immobilization until healing occurs. A figure-8 clavicular strap can be used, but simply pinning the arm to the clothing is usually sufficient. Clavicular fractures are the most common birth-trauma-related fractures. Symptoms include pain when the arm is moved. In some cases, the infant may not move the arm, especially if nerve damage has occurred. The shoulder on the affected side may appear slightly inferior to the other.

115. C: A newborn is classified as small for gestation age (SGA) if the weight is less than the 10th percentile for the newborn's age. SGA may result from intrauterine growth restriction, maternal smoking, congenital malformations, fetal infections, inadequate placental function, and chromosomal abnormalities. SGA newborns are at increased risk of meconium aspiration, polycythemia, Infants who are both preterm and SGA have increased risk. SGA newborns may be small overall or may be of normal length but have less than normal body mass.

116. B: A common probe placement for a supine infant is over the liver. The probe should not be placed over a bony area or an area with abundant brown adipose tissue, such as around the neck, the mid-scapular region of the back, the mediastinum, and organs in the thoracic cavity, kidneys, and adrenal glands. If the probe makes poor skin contact, it will indicate that the infant is cold, and the warmer will deliver increased amounts of heat, possibly causing hyperthermia. If the probe is underneath the infant, it may indicate an artificially warm temperature and decrease heat to the infant, causing hypothermia.

117. B: Distribution: The volume of distribution is the relationship between the total loading dose of drug administered and the serum concentration. (Volume of body fluid required to dissolve the amount of drug found in the serum). **Absorption:** This relates to the rate at which a drug enters the blood stream and the amount of drug. **Clearance:** Elimination pathways (liver, kidney) can become saturated if dose of medications is too high or administration is too frequent. Ideally, a drug concentration should be maintained at a steady state (average).

118. A: The three primary nutrients of human milk are carbohydrates, fat, and protein:

- Carbohydrates (40% of total calories).
- Fat (free fatty acids).
- Protein (whey to casein ratio of 60:40 and also includes IgM, IgG, lactoferrin, lysozyme, and fibronectin).

Secondary nutrients include nucleotides, vitamins (A, C, D, E), enzymes (including lipase to break down fats), growth factors, hormones (prolactin, cortisol, thyroxine, insulin, and erythropoietin), and cells (B-lymphocytes, macrophages, neutrophils, T-lymphocytes, cytokines, and interleukin 1b, 6, 8, 10, and 12.

119. C: A normal finding when assessing a neonate's fontanels is that the fontanels are level with the skull. The infant's fontanels (anterior and posterior) are covered by thick membranous tissue and should feel flat but firm. Bulging above the level of the skull may indicate increased intracranial pressure and must be reported immediately to the physician. If the fontanels are below the level of the skull, this may be an indication that the neonate is dehydrated.

120. B: Respiratory acidosis is characterized by hypoventilation and CO_2 retention along with compensatory retention of bicarbonate and increased excretion of hydrogen. Serum pH and PCO_2 are increased and urine pH is greater than 6 if compensated. Bicarbonate is increased if compensated but may be normal if uncompensated. Symptoms can include drowsiness, dizziness, headache, disorientation, seizures, and coma. Cardiac effects include flushing, ventricular fibrillation, and hypotension. Hypoventilation with hypoxia is evident.

121. B: The method of feeding that poses the fewest problems for a newborn with cleft lip and palate is bottle feeding. Most newborns with cleft lip and palate can manage to suck and some may be able to breastfeed but creating the negative pressure necessary for breastfeeding is difficult. The mother must seal the cleft with her finger or breast during breastfeeding. If the cleft is bilateral, breastfeeding may be impossible, but the mother can express milk for the infant. Some newborns may require enteral feedings in order to achieve adequate nutritional intake.

122. A: A contraindication to breastfeeding is maternal HIV positive status because the virus can be transmitted in human milk. Other contraindications include if the mother is abusing drugs, has untreated TB, or has herpes simplex lesions on a breast (although the infant can still nurse on the opposite unaffected breast). Breastfeeding may be contraindicated with some treatments, such as antimetabolites and chemotherapeutic agents. Exposure to radioactive materials also precludes breastfeeding.

123. C: Compensated metabolic acidosis is characterized by decreased serum pH, decreased PCO_2, and decreased bicarbonate. Urine pH is less than 6 when compensated. Symptoms may include drowsiness, confusion, headache, and coma. Hypotension, dysrhythmias, and flushing of skin may occur. Gastrointestinal effects can include nausea, vomiting, abdominal pain, and diarrhea. Tachypnea may be present. Causes of metabolic acidosis include diarrhea, malnutrition, and shock.

124. B: During lactation, a woman usually requires an additional 500 calories per day, generally as part of a well-balanced nutritious diet of 2500 to 2800 calories daily. However, a woman who is overweight may not need to increase caloric intake, so diet should be individualized. The woman should avoid large meals but have three smaller meals with two to three snacks. Most foods do not cause a problem for the infant, but if the infant experiences increased gas or diarrhea, it may be related to maternal diet.

125. B: Erythromycin ointment, used as a prophylaxis against ophthalmia neonatorum, should be administered into the newborn's eyes as soon as possible after birth and within one hour. Erythromycin ointment is applied to each eye in a thin strip starting from the inner canthus to the outer with excess ointment wiped away rather than washed. Silver nitrate is now rarely used because it is more irritating to the eye. Tetracycline ointment may also be used for prophylaxis.

126. C: If a woman who is breastfeeding asks when to start providing supplementary feedings, the woman should be advised to wait for at least 6 months. The American Academy of Pediatricians recommends that newborns receive only human milk for the first 6 months of life unless supplementation is medically necessary, such as if a mother is ill or the infant must be separated from the mother. In rare cases, human milk is inadequate for the infant's needs and supplementary formula may be recommended.

127. A: During resuscitation of a distressed hypoxic, bradycardic neonate, the compression-ventilation ratio should be 3:1 (90 to 30) with the compressions and ventilations administered

124

sequentially to facilitate adequate ventilation of the lungs. The compression rate should be at the rate of 120 compressions per minute with ventilations of 0.5 second. Ventilation is generally begun with room air (21% oxygen concentration and 30% for preterm infants) and oxygen titrated up if oxygen saturation is inadequate. Oxygen saturation is usually monitored on the infant's right wrist or hand.

128. A: Colostrum, which is produced by the breast for the first 2 to 4 days, serves to provide passive immunity to the neonate through high levels of immunoglobulins (antibodies). Although colostrum, which is thick and buttery in appearance, is produced in low volume (teaspoons), it is three times higher in protein (because of antibodies) than mature milk and lower in fats and carbohydrates and is adequate for the small stomach of the neonate. Colostrum also has laxative action and promotes passage of meconium.

129. B: When an infant is resuscitated using a bag and mask, air is inadvertently pumped into the stomach as it is being pumped into the lungs, so gastric suctioning is necessary. Once respirations have been stabilized either spontaneously or with mechanical ventilation, the stomach should be aspirated to remove any air pumped into it. If the air is left in the abdomen, it causes there to be an upward pressure on the lungs from the distended abdomen. This compromises lung capacity and breathing effort.

130. C: The mother should increase nursing frequency to every 2 to 3 hours, nursing until tissue softens. If the areola is taut, some milk should be manually expressed before the baby latches on. Breast pumping may make engorgement worse but may be used briefly to soften the areola. Cold compresses applied to the breasts after nursing may relieve discomfort. Engorgement almost always recedes in 24 to 48 hours, so the nurse should encourage the mother to continue breastfeeding.

131. B: When treating a neonate with hyperbilirubinemia with phototherapy, the lights should be above the neonate at a distance of 15 to 20 cm. The lights usually consist of one tungsten halogen lamp or 4-8 white or blue fluorescent lights and a Plexiglas® shield. The infant is placed under these lights with a protective mask covering the eyes to prevent retinal toxicity. The lights convert bilirubin into a water-soluble compound that can be excreted by the liver into bile and eventually into the infant's stool. The neonate should be clad only in a diaper in order to allow as much skin exposure as possible.

132. A: The mother should be questioned about her nursing technique and frequency and observed while nursing the child. Since this is her first child, she may need further assistance in nursing properly to ensure the infant receives adequate nutrition. While further tests may be indicated, these signs are indicative of dehydration and poor nutrition, so that should be dealt with first. As there are no other indications of neglect, referral to child protective services is not appropriate at this time. Switching from human milk to formula is rarely necessary if mothers receive adequate support and instruction.

133. C: If a female neonate is born with cystic hygroma (fluid-filled webbing) of the neck, swelling of distal extremities, low-set ears, and widely-spaced nipples, the neonate should be further evaluated for Turner syndrome, a genetic disorder that results from a random mutation. Other physical characteristics include cubitus valgus (elbow deformity), genu valgum (knock-knees), low posterior hairline, multiple nevi, nail dysplasia, retrognathia, ophthalmic disorders, and short stature.

134. B: Unfortified formulas (and most human milk) supply 20 calories per ounce. To ingest 120 cal/kg/day, an infant needs to ingest 6 ounces/kg/day of unfortified formula or human milk. The general requirements for adequate growth include:

- Full term infant: 100 to 120 cal/kg/day.
- Premature infants: 110 to 160 cal/kg/day.
- Infants who are recovering from surgery or have a chronic illness, such as bronchopulmonary dysplasia (BPD): ≤180 cal/kg/day.

The caloric needs of a neonate (pre-term or term) depend on postnatal age, activity, current weight, growth rate, thermal environment, and route of nutritional intake. Cold stress increases caloric requirements.

135. B: Medications that should always be included as part of the minimum neonatal resuscitation equipment include epinephrine and naloxone. Epinephrine is the AHA recommended pharmacologic intervention in the case of ineffective CPR in neonatal resuscitation. Naloxone is indicated in the case of respiratory distress in infants with opioid withdraw after the administrations of opioids as pain control in the labor process. Surfactant (indicated in respiratory distress, particularly in preterm neonates) and prostaglandins (indicated for cyanotic congenital heart defects) are useful in specific cases, but are not part of the minimum resuscitation equipment.

136. C: To reduce the risk of hemorrhagic disease after birth, a neonate should receive vitamin K. Neonates are born with low levels of vitamin K, which is necessary to activate clotting factors. Additionally, while platelet levels are near adult level, the platelets do not respond effectively to stimuli for several days after birth. Combined, these factors increase the risk of hemorrhage, but this risk is markedly reduced if the neonate receives an IM injection of vitamin K.

137. A: To facilitate bonding between the woman and her neonate if the woman chooses to bottle feed, the nurse should encourage the woman to maintain eye contact with the neonate during feedings. Maintaining skin-to-skin contact while feeding also helps to promote bonding. Holding the infant with the head higher than the body helps to prevent the child from aspirating and decreases risk of subsequent ear infections.

138. B: If a woman admitted in labor plans to relinquish her infant for adoption, the nurse should acknowledge the adoption plans: "I understand the adoptive parents have been notified that you are in labor." Broaching the subject in a supportive manner allows the mother to express feelings about the adoption if she chooses to do so. It's unlikely that little else is on the woman's mind, so pretending otherwise only isolates the woman and her feelings.

139. A: Electrolytes of primary concern in the neonate are calcium, sodium and potassium.

Electrolyte	Normal value	Discussion
Calcium	**Cord:** 8.2-11.2 mg/dL **0-10 days:** 17.6-10.4 mg/dL **11 days-2 years:** 9.0-11.0 mg/dL	**Hypocalcemia:** <7 mg/dL is common with infants that are critically ill, IDM, suffered from asphyxia, or are preterm with very low birth weight.
		Hypercalcemia: >12 mg/dL may occur with fat necrosis, congenital cardiac defects, SVA, and incorrectly mixed formula.
Sodium	Neonate: 133-146 mEq/L	**Hypernatremia:** >150 mEq/L usually relates to dehydration, use of Na containing solutions, congenital or acquired reduction in ADH, cerebral palsy, and intracranial hemorrhage.
		Hyponatremia: <130 mEq/L usually relates to overhydration, renal excretion from diuresis, or SIADH.
Potassium	Neonate: 2.7-5.9 mEq/L	**Hyperkalemia:** >7 mEq/L may relate to renal failure, acidosis, or adrenal insufficiency.
		Hypokalemia: <3.5 mEq/L usually relates to excessive GI or renal fluid losses.

140. C: If a neonate exposed to heroin during fetal development has episodes of high-pitched frantic crying comfort measure may include decreased environmental stimuli (low lights, low sound), swaddling, and rocking slowly and rhythmically or holding the neonate close to the body. Non-nutritive sucking or sucking with a sucrose-dipped pacifier may provide some relief if allowed, especially if the child sucks frantically. Playing soft music in the background may help to distract from other noises.

141. B: A total score of ≥7 is a sign of good health. APGAR is a quick evaluation of a newborn's physical condition to determine if emergency medical care is needed and is administered 1 minute and 5 minutes after birth. The highest possible score is 10.

Sign	0	1	2
Appearance (Skin Color)	Cyanotic or pallor over entire body	Normal, except for the extremities	Entire body normal
Pulse (Heart Rate)	Absent	<100 bpm	>100 bpm
Grimace (Reflex Irritability)	Unresponsive	Grimace	Infant sneezes, coughs, and recoils
Activity (Muscle Tone)	Absent	Flexed limbs	Infant moves freely
Respiration (Breathing Rate and Effort)	Absent	Bradypnea, dyspnea	Good breathing and crying

142. C: If, when a new mother is trying to breastfeed, the neonate latches on to just the nipple, the nurse should advise the mother to insert a finger at the side of the infant's mouth to break the suction and to start over. The nipple must extend into the infant's mouth to the soft palate because if it ends at the hard palate, the suckling movements will result in irritation and discomfort.

143. A: If a nursing neonate has a 5:1 suck/swallow ratio, this indicates non-nutritive suckling. The normal suck/swallow ratio is 2:1 or 1:1, which indicates that an adequate volume of milk is being obtained. If the suck/swallow ratio is 5:1 or greater, the neonate is probably getting very little or no

127

milk and may become exhausted from trying to suckle, and the milk supply will decrease because of inadequate stimulation of the breast. The woman may need assistance from a breastfeeding specialist.

144. C: A neonate should no longer exhibit head lag with the pull-to-site test by age 4 months. If head lag persists beyond 4 months, then the infant needs further neurological evaluation. For the pull-to-sit test, the neonate should begin in the supine position and pulled slowly to sitting position by grasping and pulling on the arms. After birth, the head generally lags behind trunk, but the neck should not be completely flexed backward. The neonate can usually pull the head forward when in sitting position for brief periods even though the head may be wobbly.

145. C: If a neonate had necrotizing enterocolitis, resulting in removal of a significant portion of the jejunum and short gut/bowel syndrome, the neonate is likely to have malabsorption of calories, proteins, carbohydrates, and fats, especially if the remaining portion of the jejunum is less than 100 cm in length. Removal of significant portions of the ileum results in steatorrhea and poor absorption of fat-soluble vitamins (K, A, D, E) and vitamin B12. Over time, the small bowel grows in length and adapts, increasing absorption.

146. A: Current discharge requirement are based on physiological and functional readiness. Requirements generally include:

- The infant is feeding appropriately, as evidenced by:
  - Primary caregiver feeding the infant with the prescribed method (gavage, gastrostomy, or special positioning) consistently.
  - Weight gain of 15-30 grams per day over several days.
- Feeds accomplished without respiratory difficulty.
- All medical or surgical problems that require hospitalization are resolved.
- Temperature stability is maintained in an open crib.
- Parents are trained appropriately concerning administration of medications, CPR, and proper use of car seat.
- Infant has passed all pre-discharge tests:
- Age appropriate immunizations were administered.

147. B: If a neonate begins to bob the head and bring the hands to the mouth, this probably indicates hunger and is a feeding cue. Signs of hunger may be subtle with crying (squawking) typically the last sign. Once an infant begins crying and frantic, the child may have difficulty latching on. Other signs of hunger include licking, sucking motions, rooting, bringing hands to mouth or face, and trying to suck a finger stroking the infant's cheek or lower lip. If the neonate is consistently underfed, the infant may become listless and show less interest in nursing.

148. C: The pain control measure that is appropriate for a newborn that has just had a circumcision is acetaminophen. Codeine is not recommended for newborns because of impaired metabolism of opioids and because pain should not be severe after circumcision. Acetaminophen is well-tolerated in appropriate doses. Aspirin should be avoided in infants and small children because of the risk of Reye's syndrome if the newborn has a viral infection and takes aspirin. Oral sucrose is often administered prior to the procedure to minimize the pain accompanying it.

149. B: The vaccination that should be routinely administered to all newborns within 24 hours of birth is hepatitis B. The second dose should be given within the first to second month and the third dose between 6 and 18 months. If the neonate's mother is hepatitis B positive, then the neonate should receive the vaccination within 12 hours of birth and 0.5 mL of hepatitis B immune globulin

(HBIG). If the mother's status is unknown, the neonate should also receive the vaccination within 12 hours of birth and the mother tested.

150. A: When facilitating quality improvement, the biggest barrier to implementation of changes is usually staff resistance to change. People develop a sense of security with familiarity, and new approaches, even though they may be demonstrably better, can result in anxiety and insecurity. Some people may feel that the changes suggests that they were less than competent before, and others may resent the time and effort needed to learn new skills or ways of doing things.

151. B: A newborn should normally breastfeed between 8 to 12 times in 24 hours (every 1 to 3 hours). The woman should begin breastfeeding on the last breast used at the previous feeding. Infants usually nurse for 15 to 20 minutes on each side during each feeding. If nursing times are appreciably shorter or longer, then the woman may need counseling from a lactation specialist to determine the reason. Women should be advised that infants may feed more frequently during growth spurts that occur at 2 to 3 weeks, 6 weeks, 3 months, and 6 months.

152. C: Normal term neonate skin appearance at birth should include deep cracks, no visible blood vessels, and little vernix. When skin develops during week 15 of gestation, it is initially thin and translucent. By week 20, vernix caseosa production begins. The stratum corneum (top epidermal layer) develops from weeks 20-24. The epidermis continues to develop and thicken and forms a water barrier by week 32. Near term, the vernix washes away and the skin becomes more wrinkled without its protection.

153. B: When levels of estrogen and progesterone decrease in the postpartal period, this causes the anterior pituitary gland to produce increased levels of prolactin to prepare for lactation. The increase is especially marked in the first postpartal week but then falls about 50%, although still elevated above normal rates. If the woman chooses not to breastfeed, then the levels of prolactin decrease and are usually back to normal non-pregnant levels by the end of a week.

154. B: Freshly expressed human milk can be stored at room temperature for 4 hours or kept in the refrigerator for 5 to 7 days at a temperature ranging from 34 to 39° F (1 to 4° C). Human milk can also be kept frozen for 6 to 12 months at temperatures of 0° F (-19° C). If possible, a woman should pump the breasts and save the milk every time a feeding is missed, but that may not be possible if the woman is employed. In that case, the woman should pump at least two times in an 8-hour shift.

155. C: Following birth, an infant of a diabetic mother (IDM) is at greatest risk of hypoglycemia at 0.5 to 1.5 hours. The fetus increases production of insulin around 20 weeks of gestation in response to the mother's elevated blood glucose. When the umbilical cord is cut, it abruptly disrupts the neonate's supply of glucose while the insulin level remains elevated. The neonate may have increased glucose need for several days to prevent hypoglycemia (as high as 10 to 15 mg/kg/min).

156. B: If a neonate is diagnosed with galactosemia through routine newborn metabolic screening, in order to prevent severe intellectual disability, the neonate must only receive lactose-free formula. Galactosemia is an autosomal recessive disorder in which the neonate lacks the enzyme that converts galactose (found in lactose) to glucose. Clinical indications include jaundice, vomiting, diarrhea, inability to gain weight and hypoglycemia. An infant that does not receive treatment can contract a serious gram-negative infection related to damage to the intestinal lining, and death may occur at 1 to 2 weeks.

157. B: If a newborn develops diaper dermatitis, the initial treatment should be to cleanse with mild soap and water, dry, and expose to the air. Baby wipes and lotions should be avoided as they may cause an allergic response. Antibiotic ointment may cause a rash. If the dermatitis is severe or draining, then this may indicate an infection and the physician should be contacted. Diapers should be changed promptly when wet and a barrier ointment or cream (such as petrolatum jelly or zinc oxide) may be applied.

158. C: While postpartum depression can occur at any time after childbirth, the most common onset is at about 4 weeks postpartum. Duration varies from about 3 months to 14 months. The woman may feel very sad and helpless and have insomnia and difficulty concentrating. Some woman may feel suicidal and/or hostile toward others, including the infant. If the woman has negative feelings toward the infant, the infant may need to be cared for by others until the woman's depression improves.

159. C: Women who are pregnant should avoid contact with cat feces because of risk of infection with toxoplasmosis, which may also be acquired through ingesting undercooked meat or unpasteurized goat's milk. Fetal risk is highest if infection occurs during the first trimester as the infection may result in microcephaly and hydrocephalus or spontaneous abortion. Mild infections may cause retinochoroiditis while severe infections may cause seizures and CNS abnormalities. If the woman becomes infected, treatment (spiramycin, pyrimethamine, sulfonamide) may reduce the severity of fetal abnormalities.

160. A: Normal vital signs for a term infant who is awake but not crying are HR 160, BP 70/44 and RR 40.

Blood pressure	56/33 to 77/50 mmHg
	Hypertension: Systolic >90 and diastolic >60.
Pulse	120-180 bpm awake
	100 bpm asleep
	180 bpm crying
	220 bpm active/sick
Respirations	30-60 per minute
Temperature	Stabilizes within 8-12 hours.
	Ranges from 36.3-37.0 °C.

161. B: If a neonate with congestive heart failure is receiving furosemide to relieve pulmonary edema, the neonate should be monitored for electrolyte imbalances because furosemide increases risk of hypokalemia, hypochloremia, and hypocalcemia. Excess calcium is lost through the kidneys and urine and may result in nephrocalcinosis (deposits of calcium in the renal parenchyma). Other diuretic options include chlorothiazide, which causes less loss of potassium and calcium, and spironolactone, which is potassium sparing but can result in hyperkalemia.

162. A: If a neonate with DiGeorge syndrome, usually resulting from a deletion on chromosome 22 (22q11.2), has severe immunocompromise as indicated by an exceptionally low T-lymphocyte count, this is an indication of thymus abnormality or absence. The infant is at severe risk of infection. Other abnormalities associated with DiGeorge syndrome include hypocalcemia, congenital heart disease (usually involving the aorta), and facial abnormalities (micrognathia, abnormal placement and structure of ears, and heavy eyelids). The neonate is also at risk for other autoimmune diseases, such as Hashimoto's thyroiditis and ITP.

163. C: Inadequate or poor handwashing technique is one of the most common causes of the infant-to-infant spread of infection in hospitals. Hands should be washed before and after every patient contact or when removing gloves. Handwashing should be done under running water with plain soap, scrubbing the hands, nails, and wrists thoroughly, and the faucet turned off by using the elbow, upper arm, or paper towel. Alcohol-based rubs used for hand disinfection (at least 15 seconds) are effective against *Staphylococcus aureus* but are not effective against *Clostridium difficile.*

164. B: If a male newborn has hypospadias (a congenital defect where the urethra opens onto the underside of the penis and not in its usual place at the tip), the neonate should be carefully examined for undescended testicles and inguinal hernia as these are the most common anomalies found in association with hypospadias. The neonate may also have chordee (curvature) of the penis. Surgical repair is usually indicated but is not emergent if the neonate is urinating without difficulty. Circumcision should be delayed as some tissue from the prepuce may be utilized during repair.

165. B: The sexually-transmitted disease that can infect the fetus and cause the multiple system disorders in the neonate, including non-viral hepatitis, hepatosplenomegaly, myocarditis, palmer/plantar rash, and bone marrow failure, is syphilis. The neonate may also develop meningitis, anemia, and edema associated with nephritic syndrome. Some infants may be asymptomatic at birth even with severe infection but will develop symptoms later. Maternal trichomonas infection may result in preterm birth and low birth weight. Chlamydia may cause conjunctivitis.

166. C: Retinopathy of prematurity is associated with hyperoxia. ROP is an abnormal vascular proliferative disease of the immature retina and is associated with infants born ≤31 week and <1500 g (50-70% of infants whose birth weight is <1,250 grams). Retinal vascularization begins at around 16 weeks' gestation and completes at full term. Premature birth interrupts this normal progression. Exposure of these infants to hyperoxia causes reduction in their production of retinal vascular endothelial growth factor and vasoconstriction, which causes the retina to thicken, resulting in hypoxia that, in turn, triggers disorganized growth of new blood vessels and scarring.

167. A: If a mother is blood type O and the fetus type A or B, the neonate may develop hyperbilirubinemia although complications are usually not serious. In rare instances, hemolysis may be severe enough to require exchange transfusions. The rate of breakdown of red blood cells increases, so the neonate may be at risk for anemia in the weeks after delivery, so the neonate's blood counts should be monitored. ABO incompatibility occurs in about 20% to 25% of pregnancies.

168. B: During the neonate's physical assessment for the Babinski reflex, stroking the lateral aspect of the sole of the foot from the heel to the ball of the foot should elicit hyperextension (fanning) of the toes because the neonate's neurological system is not fully developed. The Babinski reflex is normal for the first one to two years of life but is pathological after that time, indicating neurological compromise. The Babinski reflex is recorded as being present or absent.

169. A: if a neonate with spina bifida exhibits slight bulging of the fontanels and distended scalp veins, these are early signs of hydrocephalus, a common complication of neural tube defects. Hydrocephalus occurs with imbalance between production and absorption of cerebrospinal fluid. Treatment includes insertion of ventriculoperitoneal shunt. In some cases, hydrocephalus may also be caused by intraventricular hemorrhage, but symptoms are usually more severe and can occur rapidly because of increasing intracranial pressure.

170. C: A female neonate with congenital hyperplasia, an autosomal recessive defect, will most likely have enlarged clitoris or male-appearing genitalia. In some cases, the genitalia may appear ambiguous; for example, the labia may be fused, giving the appearance of a scrotum but without evidence of testes. The gender of the child may not be immediately clear at birth. Because the fetus was exposed to masculinizing hormones during development, the neonate may eventually identify more with the male gender than female.

171. A: If a neonate shows a sudden drop of platelet count from 200,000 to 50,000 four days after birth, the most likely cause is sepsis. Late-onset neonatal thrombocytopenia occurs after three days, and if the rate falls to below 50,000, the infant may be at risk of hemorrhage although the benefits of platelet transfusions is not established with levels above 20,000 unless the neonate is actively hemorrhaging. Neonates with early onset thrombocytopenia and are preterm <28 weeks are particularly at risk for hemorrhage and should receive transfusion if levels fall below 30,000.

172. B: If a neonate must have a transfusion with packed red blood cells, it should be given in increments of 15 to 20 mL/kg to prevent overhydration. This volume increases the hemoglobin by 2 to 3 g/L. Benefits of the transfusion include relief of anemia and improved oxygenation. PRBCs are often preferred over whole blood because of the reduced volume. Risks associated with transfusions include infection, transfusion reaction (rare), GVHD, and fluid overload.

173. C: The only immunoglobulin that can cross the placenta is IgG. IgG is the primary immunoglobulin found in serum (comprises 75% of immunoglobulins) and extravascular areas and has a major role in the immune response because it is the most versatile. IgM have an important role in agglutinating pathogens so they can be removed from the body. IgA in found in secretions (such as tears and mucus) and has a role in mucosal immunity.

174. B: Insensible water losses (IWL) occur as water evaporates from the skin (2/3) or the respiratory tract (1/3). IWL cannot be directly measured. Premature neonates have thin skin that allows for increased amounts of evaporative water loss. As the skin matures and the stratum corneum develops (around 31 weeks of gestation) less water is lost through the skin. A full-term neonate will have an IWL of 12/ml/kg/24 hours at 50% humidity. Factors that increase IWL include prematurity, radiant warmers, phototherapy, fever, low humidity, and tachypnea. Sensible water losses occur via urination, stool, and gastric drainage and can be accurately measured.

175. C: Mastitis causes induration, swelling, erythema, increasing fever, acute pain, and sometimes painful abscesses. The infected area may be localized or generalized. The mother may have chills and flu-like symptoms before obvious inflammation of the breast. Usually the mother becomes infected from the infant (generally *Staphylococcus aureus*) so breastfeeding does not endanger the neonate. Treatment includes antibiotics (usually penicillin G, dicloxacillin, or erythromycin) and nursing (or pumping or expressing) on the affected side to prevent abscess formation. Applying heat or massaging the breasts in a warm shower may increase circulation. Pain relief includes alternating warm and cold compresses and acetaminophen or ibuprofen.

How to Overcome Test Anxiety

Just the thought of taking a test is enough to make most people a little nervous. A test is an important event that can have a long-term impact on your future, so it's important to take it seriously and it's natural to feel anxious about performing well. But just because anxiety is normal, that doesn't mean that it's helpful in test taking, or that you should simply accept it as part of your life. Anxiety can have a variety of effects. These effects can be mild, like making you feel slightly nervous, or severe, like blocking your ability to focus or remember even a simple detail.

If you experience test anxiety—whether severe or mild—it's important to know how to beat it. To discover this, first you need to understand what causes test anxiety.

Causes of Test Anxiety

While we often think of anxiety as an uncontrollable emotional state, it can actually be caused by simple, practical things. One of the most common causes of test anxiety is that a person does not feel adequately prepared for their test. This feeling can be the result of many different issues such as poor study habits or lack of organization, but the most common culprit is time management. Starting to study too late, failing to organize your study time to cover all of the material, or being distracted while you study will mean that you're not well prepared for the test. This may lead to cramming the night before, which will cause you to be physically and mentally exhausted for the test. Poor time management also contributes to feelings of stress, fear, and hopelessness as you realize you are not well prepared but don't know what to do about it.

Other times, test anxiety is not related to your preparation for the test but comes from unresolved fear. This may be a past failure on a test, or poor performance on tests in general. It may come from comparing yourself to others who seem to be performing better or from the stress of living up to expectations. Anxiety may be driven by fears of the future—how failure on this test would affect your educational and career goals. These fears are often completely irrational, but they can still negatively impact your test performance.

> **Review Video: 3 Reasons You Have Test Anxiety**
> Visit mometrix.com/academy and enter code: 428468

133

Elements of Test Anxiety

As mentioned earlier, test anxiety is considered to be an emotional state, but it has physical and mental components as well. Sometimes you may not even realize that you are suffering from test anxiety until you notice the physical symptoms. These can include trembling hands, rapid heartbeat, sweating, nausea, and tense muscles. Extreme anxiety may lead to fainting or vomiting. Obviously, any of these symptoms can have a negative impact on testing. It is important to recognize them as soon as they begin to occur so that you can address the problem before it damages your performance.

> **Review Video: 3 Ways to Tell You Have Test Anxiety**
> Visit mometrix.com/academy and enter code: 927847

The mental components of test anxiety include trouble focusing and inability to remember learned information. During a test, your mind is on high alert, which can help you recall information and stay focused for an extended period of time. However, anxiety interferes with your mind's natural processes, causing you to blank out, even on the questions you know well. The strain of testing during anxiety makes it difficult to stay focused, especially on a test that may take several hours. Extreme anxiety can take a huge mental toll, making it difficult not only to recall test information but even to understand the test questions or pull your thoughts together.

> **Review Video: How Test Anxiety Affects Memory**
> Visit mometrix.com/academy and enter code: 609003

Effects of Test Anxiety

Test anxiety is like a disease—if left untreated, it will get progressively worse. Anxiety leads to poor performance, and this reinforces the feelings of fear and failure, which in turn lead to poor performances on subsequent tests. It can grow from a mild nervousness to a crippling condition. If allowed to progress, test anxiety can have a big impact on your schooling, and consequently on your future.

Test anxiety can spread to other parts of your life. Anxiety on tests can become anxiety in any stressful situation, and blanking on a test can turn into panicking in a job situation. But fortunately, you don't have to let anxiety rule your testing and determine your grades. There are a number of relatively simple steps you can take to move past anxiety and function normally on a test and in the rest of life.

> **Review Video: How Test Anxiety Impacts Your Grades**
> Visit mometrix.com/academy and enter code: 939819

Physical Steps for Beating Test Anxiety

While test anxiety is a serious problem, the good news is that it can be overcome. It doesn't have to control your ability to think and remember information. While it may take time, you can begin taking steps today to beat anxiety.

Just as your first hint that you may be struggling with anxiety comes from the physical symptoms, the first step to treating it is also physical. Rest is crucial for having a clear, strong mind. If you are tired, it is much easier to give in to anxiety. But if you establish good sleep habits, your body and mind will be ready to perform optimally, without the strain of exhaustion. Additionally, sleeping well helps you to retain information better, so you're more likely to recall the answers when you see the test questions.

Getting good sleep means more than going to bed on time. It's important to allow your brain time to relax. Take study breaks from time to time so it doesn't get overworked, and don't study right before bed. Take time to rest your mind before trying to rest your body, or you may find it difficult to fall asleep.

> **Review Video: <u>The Importance of Sleep for Your Brain</u>**
> Visit mometrix.com/academy and enter code: 319338

Along with sleep, other aspects of physical health are important in preparing for a test. Good nutrition is vital for good brain function. Sugary foods and drinks may give a burst of energy but this burst is followed by a crash, both physically and emotionally. Instead, fuel your body with protein and vitamin-rich foods.

Also, drink plenty of water. Dehydration can lead to headaches and exhaustion, especially if your brain is already under stress from the rigors of the test. Particularly if your test is a long one, drink water during the breaks. And if possible, take an energy-boosting snack to eat between sections.

> **Review Video: <u>How Diet Can Affect your Mood</u>**
> Visit mometrix.com/academy and enter code: 624317

Along with sleep and diet, a third important part of physical health is exercise. Maintaining a steady workout schedule is helpful, but even taking 5-minute study breaks to walk can help get your blood pumping faster and clear your head. Exercise also releases endorphins, which contribute to a positive feeling and can help combat test anxiety.

When you nurture your physical health, you are also contributing to your mental health. If your body is healthy, your mind is much more likely to be healthy as well. So take time to rest, nourish your body with healthy food and water, and get moving as much as possible. Taking these physical steps will make you stronger and more able to take the mental steps necessary to overcome test anxiety.

> **Review Video: <u>How to Stay Healthy and Prevent Test Anxiety</u>**
> Visit mometrix.com/academy and enter code: 877894

Mental Steps for Beating Test Anxiety

Working on the mental side of test anxiety can be more challenging, but as with the physical side, there are clear steps you can take to overcome it. As mentioned earlier, test anxiety often stems from lack of preparation, so the obvious solution is to prepare for the test. Effective studying may be the most important weapon you have for beating test anxiety, but you can and should employ several other mental tools to combat fear.

First, boost your confidence by reminding yourself of past success—tests or projects that you aced. If you're putting as much effort into preparing for this test as you did for those, there's no reason you should expect to fail here. Work hard to prepare; then trust your preparation.

Second, surround yourself with encouraging people. It can be helpful to find a study group, but be sure that the people you're around will encourage a positive attitude. If you spend time with others who are anxious or cynical, this will only contribute to your own anxiety. Look for others who are motivated to study hard from a desire to succeed, not from a fear of failure.

Third, reward yourself. A test is physically and mentally tiring, even without anxiety, and it can be helpful to have something to look forward to. Plan an activity following the test, regardless of the outcome, such as going to a movie or getting ice cream.

When you are taking the test, if you find yourself beginning to feel anxious, remind yourself that you know the material. Visualize successfully completing the test. Then take a few deep, relaxing breaths and return to it. Work through the questions carefully but with confidence, knowing that you are capable of succeeding.

Developing a healthy mental approach to test taking will also aid in other areas of life. Test anxiety affects more than just the actual test—it can be damaging to your mental health and even contribute to depression. It's important to beat test anxiety before it becomes a problem for more than testing.

> **Review Video: Test Anxiety and Depression**
> Visit mometrix.com/academy and enter code: 904704

Study Strategy

Being prepared for the test is necessary to combat anxiety, but what does being prepared look like? You may study for hours on end and still not feel prepared. What you need is a strategy for test prep. The next few pages outline our recommended steps to help you plan out and conquer the challenge of preparation.

STEP 1: SCOPE OUT THE TEST

Learn everything you can about the format (multiple choice, essay, etc.) and what will be on the test. Gather any study materials, course outlines, or sample exams that may be available. Not only will this help you to prepare, but knowing what to expect can help to alleviate test anxiety.

STEP 2: MAP OUT THE MATERIAL

Look through the textbook or study guide and make note of how many chapters or sections it has. Then divide these over the time you have. For example, if a book has 15 chapters and you have five days to study, you need to cover three chapters each day. Even better, if you have the time, leave an extra day at the end for overall review after you have gone through the material in depth.

If time is limited, you may need to prioritize the material. Look through it and make note of which sections you think you already have a good grasp on, and which need review. While you are studying, skim quickly through the familiar sections and take more time on the challenging parts. Write out your plan so you don't get lost as you go. Having a written plan also helps you feel more in control of the study, so anxiety is less likely to arise from feeling overwhelmed at the amount to cover.

STEP 3: GATHER YOUR TOOLS

Decide what study method works best for you. Do you prefer to highlight in the book as you study and then go back over the highlighted portions? Or do you type out notes of the important information? Or is it helpful to make flashcards that you can carry with you? Assemble the pens, index cards, highlighters, post-it notes, and any other materials you may need so you won't be distracted by getting up to find things while you study.

If you're having a hard time retaining the information or organizing your notes, experiment with different methods. For example, try color-coding by subject with colored pens, highlighters, or post-it notes. If you learn better by hearing, try recording yourself reading your notes so you can listen while in the car, working out, or simply sitting at your desk. Ask a friend to quiz you from your flashcards, or try teaching someone the material to solidify it in your mind.

STEP 4: CREATE YOUR ENVIRONMENT

It's important to avoid distractions while you study. This includes both the obvious distractions like visitors and the subtle distractions like an uncomfortable chair (or a too-comfortable couch that makes you want to fall asleep). Set up the best study environment possible: good lighting and a comfortable work area. If background music helps you focus, you may want to turn it on, but otherwise keep the room quiet. If you are using a computer to take notes, be sure you don't have any other windows open, especially applications like social media, games, or anything else that could distract you. Silence your phone and turn off notifications. Be sure to keep water close by so you stay hydrated while you study (but avoid unhealthy drinks and snacks).

Also, take into account the best time of day to study. Are you freshest first thing in the morning? Try to set aside some time then to work through the material. Is your mind clearer in the afternoon or evening? Schedule your study session then. Another method is to study at the same time of day that you will take the test, so that your brain gets used to working on the material at that time and will be ready to focus at test time.

STEP 5: STUDY!

Once you have done all the study preparation, it's time to settle into the actual studying. Sit down, take a few moments to settle your mind so you can focus, and begin to follow your study plan. Don't give in to distractions or let yourself procrastinate. This is your time to prepare so you'll be ready to fearlessly approach the test. Make the most of the time and stay focused.

Of course, you don't want to burn out. If you study too long you may find that you're not retaining the information very well. Take regular study breaks. For example, taking five minutes out of every hour to walk briskly, breathing deeply and swinging your arms, can help your mind stay fresh.

As you get to the end of each chapter or section, it's a good idea to do a quick review. Remind yourself of what you learned and work on any difficult parts. When you feel that you've mastered the material, move on to the next part. At the end of your study session, briefly skim through your notes again.

But while review is helpful, cramming last minute is NOT. If at all possible, work ahead so that you won't need to fit all your study into the last day. Cramming overloads your brain with more information than it can process and retain, and your tired mind may struggle to recall even previously learned information when it is overwhelmed with last-minute study. Also, the urgent nature of cramming and the stress placed on your brain contribute to anxiety. You'll be more likely to go to the test feeling unprepared and having trouble thinking clearly.

So don't cram, and don't stay up late before the test, even just to review your notes at a leisurely pace. Your brain needs rest more than it needs to go over the information again. In fact, plan to finish your studies by noon or early afternoon the day before the test. Give your brain the rest of the day to relax or focus on other things, and get a good night's sleep. Then you will be fresh for the test and better able to recall what you've studied.

STEP 6: TAKE A PRACTICE TEST

Many courses offer sample tests, either online or in the study materials. This is an excellent resource to check whether you have mastered the material, as well as to prepare for the test format and environment.

Check the test format ahead of time: the number of questions, the type (multiple choice, free response, etc.), and the time limit. Then create a plan for working through them. For example, if you have 30 minutes to take a 60-question test, your limit is 30 seconds per question. Spend less time on the questions you know well so that you can take more time on the difficult ones.

If you have time to take several practice tests, take the first one open book, with no time limit. Work through the questions at your own pace and make sure you fully understand them. Gradually work up to taking a test under test conditions: sit at a desk with all study materials put away and set a timer. Pace yourself to make sure you finish the test with time to spare and go back to check your answers if you have time.

After each test, check your answers. On the questions you missed, be sure you understand why you missed them. Did you misread the question (tests can use tricky wording)? Did you forget the information? Or was it something you hadn't learned? Go back and study any shaky areas that the practice tests reveal.

Taking these tests not only helps with your grade, but also aids in combating test anxiety. If you're already used to the test conditions, you're less likely to worry about it, and working through tests until you're scoring well gives you a confidence boost. Go through the practice tests until you feel comfortable, and then you can go into the test knowing that you're ready for it.

Test Tips

On test day, you should be confident, knowing that you've prepared well and are ready to answer the questions. But aside from preparation, there are several test day strategies you can employ to maximize your performance.

First, as stated before, get a good night's sleep the night before the test (and for several nights before that, if possible). Go into the test with a fresh, alert mind rather than staying up late to study.

Try not to change too much about your normal routine on the day of the test. It's important to eat a nutritious breakfast, but if you normally don't eat breakfast at all, consider eating just a protein bar. If you're a coffee drinker, go ahead and have your normal coffee. Just make sure you time it so that the caffeine doesn't wear off right in the middle of your test. Avoid sugary beverages, and drink enough water to stay hydrated but not so much that you need a restroom break 10 minutes into the test. If your test isn't first thing in the morning, consider going for a walk or doing a light workout before the test to get your blood flowing.

Allow yourself enough time to get ready, and leave for the test with plenty of time to spare so you won't have the anxiety of scrambling to arrive in time. Another reason to be early is to select a good seat. It's helpful to sit away from doors and windows, which can be distracting. Find a good seat, get out your supplies, and settle your mind before the test begins.

When the test begins, start by going over the instructions carefully, even if you already know what to expect. Make sure you avoid any careless mistakes by following the directions.

Then begin working through the questions, pacing yourself as you've practiced. If you're not sure on an answer, don't spend too much time on it, and don't let it shake your confidence. Either skip it and come back later, or eliminate as many wrong answers as possible and guess among the remaining ones. Don't dwell on these questions as you continue—put them out of your mind and focus on what lies ahead.

Be sure to read all of the answer choices, even if you're sure the first one is the right answer. Sometimes you'll find a better one if you keep reading. But don't second-guess yourself if you do immediately know the answer. Your gut instinct is usually right. Don't let test anxiety rob you of the information you know.

If you have time at the end of the test (and if the test format allows), go back and review your answers. Be cautious about changing any, since your first instinct tends to be correct, but make sure you didn't misread any of the questions or accidentally mark the wrong answer choice. Look over any you skipped and make an educated guess.

At the end, leave the test feeling confident. You've done your best, so don't waste time worrying about your performance or wishing you could change anything. Instead, celebrate the successful completion of this test. And finally, use this test to learn how to deal with anxiety even better next time.

Review Video: 5 Tips to Beat Test Anxiety
Visit mometrix.com/academy and enter code: 570656

Important Qualification

Not all anxiety is created equal. If your test anxiety is causing major issues in your life beyond the classroom or testing center, or if you are experiencing troubling physical symptoms related to your anxiety, it may be a sign of a serious physiological or psychological condition. If this sounds like your situation, we strongly encourage you to seek professional help.

Thank You

We at Mometrix would like to extend our heartfelt thanks to you, our friend and patron, for allowing us to play a part in your journey. It is a privilege to serve people from all walks of life who are unified in their commitment to building the best future they can for themselves.

The preparation you devote to these important testing milestones may be the most valuable educational opportunity you have for making a real difference in your life. We encourage you to put your heart into it—that feeling of succeeding, overcoming, and yes, conquering will be well worth the hours you've invested.

We want to hear your story, your struggles and your successes, and if you see any opportunities for us to improve our materials so we can help others even more effectively in the future, please share that with us as well. **The team at Mometrix would be absolutely thrilled to hear from you!** So please, send us an email (support@mometrix.com) and let's stay in touch.

> **If you'd like some additional help, check out these other resources we offer for your exam:**
> **http://mometrixflashcards.com/Neonatal**

Additional Bonus Material

Due to our efforts to try to keep this book to a manageable length, we've created a link that will give you access to all of your additional bonus material.

Please visit **https://www.mometrix.com/bonus948/lrneonatal**
to access the information.